COGNITIVE THERAPY: BASICS AND BEYOND

COGNITIVE THERAPY: BASICS AND BEYOND

Judith S. Beck, Ph.D.

Foreword by Aaron T. Beck, M.D.

The Guilford Press
New York   London

©1995 The Guilford Press
A Division of Guilford Publications
72 Spring Street, New York, NY 10012

Printed in the United States of America

This book is printed on acid-free paper.

Last digit is print number: 9 8 7 6 5 4 3 2

Library of Congress Cataloging-in-Publication-Data

Beck, Judith S.
    Cognitive therapy :   basics and beyond / Judith S. Beck ; foreword by Aaron T. Beck.
        p.   cm.
    Includes bibliographical references and index.
    ISBN 0-89862-847-4
    1. Cognitive therapy.   I. Title.
    [DNLM: 1. Cognitive Therapy—methods. WM 425.5.C6 B393c 1995]
RC489.C63B43   1995
616.89'142—dc20
DNLM/DLC
for Library of Congress   95-12521
                                                                        CIP

To my father,
Aaron T. Beck, M.D.

FOREWORD

W hat is the purpose of this book?" is a natural question raised by the reader of any book on psychotherapy and to be addressed in the foreword. To answer this question for readers of Dr. Judith Beck's book, *Cognitive Therapy: Basics and Beyond*, I need to take the reader back to the early days of cognitive therapy and its development since then.

When I first started treating patients with a set of therapeutic procedures that I later labeled "cognitive therapy," I had no idea where this approach—which departed so strongly from my psychoanalytic training—would lead me. Based on my clinical observations and some systematic clinical studies and experiments, I theorized that there was a thinking disorder at the core of the psychiatric syndromes such as depression and anxiety. This disorder was reflected in a systematic bias in the way the patients interpreted particular experiences. By pointing out these biased interpretations and proposing alternatives—that is, more probable explanations—I found that I could produce an almost immediate lessening of the symptoms. Training the patients in these cognitive skills helped to sustain the improvement. This concentration on here-and-now problems appeared to produce almost total alleviation of symptoms in 10 to 14 weeks. Later clinical trials by my own group and clinicians/investigators elsewhere supported the efficacy of this approach for anxiety disorders, depressive disorders, and panic disorder.

By the mid-1980s, I could claim that cognitive therapy had attained the status of a "System of Psychotherapy." It consisted of (1) a theory of personality and psychopathology with solid empirical findings to support its basic postulates; (2) a model of psychotherapy, with sets of principles and strategies that blended with the theory of psychopathology; and (3) solid empirical findings based on clinical outcome studies to support the efficacy of this approach.

Since my earlier work, a new generation of therapists/researchers/teachers has conducted basic investigations of the conceptual model of psychopathology and applied cognitive therapy to a broad spectrum of psychiatric disorders. The systematic investigations explore the basic cognitive dimensions of personality and the psychiatric disorders, the idiosyncratic processing and recall of information in these disorders, and the relationship between vulnerability and stress.

The applications of cognitive therapy to a host of psychological and medical disorders extended far beyond anything I could have imagined when I treated my first few cases of depression and anxiety with cognitive therapy. On the basis of outcome trials, investigators throughout the world, but particularly the United States, have established that cognitive therapy is effective in conditions as diverse as posttraumatic stress disorder, obsessive–compulsive disorder, phobias of all kinds, and eating disorders. Often in combination with medication it has been helpful in the treatment of bipolar affective disorder and schizophrenia. Cognitive therapy has also been found to be beneficial in a wide variety of chronic medical disorders such as low back pain, colitis, hypertension, and chronic fatigue syndrome.

With a smorgasbord of applications of cognitive therapy, how can an aspiring cognitive therapist begin to learn the nuts and bolts of this therapy? Extracting from *Alice in Wonderland,* "Start at the beginning." This now brings us back to the question at the beginning of this foreword. The purpose of this book by Dr. Judith Beck, one of the new generation of cognitive therapists (and who, as a teenager, was one of the first to listen to me expound on my new theory), is to provide a solid basic foundation for the practice of cognitive therapy. Despite the formidable array of different applications of cognitive therapy, they all are based on fundamental principles outlined in this volume. Other books (some of them authored by me) have guided the cognitive therapist through the maze of each of the specific disorders. This volume will take their place, I believe, as the basic text for cognitive therapists. Even experienced cognitive therapists should find this book quite helpful in sharpening their conceptualization skills, expanding their repertoire of therapeutic techniques, planning more effective treatment, and troubleshooting difficulties in therapy.

Of course, no book can substitute for supervision in cognitive therapy. But this book is an important volume and can be supplemented by supervision, which is readily available from a network of trained cognitive therapists (Appendix D).

Dr. Judith Beck is eminently qualified to offer this guide to cognitive therapy. For the past 10 years, she has conducted workshops and case conferences and has lectured on cognitive therapy, supervised numerous beginners and experienced therapists in cognitive therapy, helped develop treatment protocols for various disorders, and participated actively in research on cognitive therapy. With such a background to draw on, she has written a book with a rich lode of information to apply this therapy.

The practice of cognitive therapy is not simple. I have observed a number of participants in clinical trials, for example, who can go through the motions of working with "automatic thoughts," without any real understanding of the patients' perceptions of their personal world or any sense of the principle of "collaborative empiricism." The purpose of Dr. Judith Beck's book is to educate, to teach, and to train both the novice and the experienced therapist in cognitive therapy, and she has succeeded admirably in this mission.

AARON T. BECK, M.D.

PREFACE

While presenting workshops and seminars both nationally and internationally over the past 10 years, I have been struck by three things. First is the growing enthusiasm for cognitive therapy, one of a very few unified systems of psychotherapy that have been empirically validated. Second is the strong desire of mental health professionals to learn how to do cognitive therapy in a consistent way, guided by a robust conceptualization and knowledge of techniques. Third is the large number of misconceptions about cognitive therapy, such as the following: that it is merely a set of techniques; that it downplays the importance of emotions and of the therapeutic relationship; and that it disregards the childhood origin of many psychological difficulties.

Countless workshop participants have told me that they have been using cognitive techniques for years, without ever labeling them as such. Others, familiar with the first manual of cognitive therapy, *Cognitive Therapy of Depression* (Beck, Rush, Shaw, & Emery, 1979), have struggled with learning to apply this form of therapy more effectively. This book is designed for a broad audience, from those mental health professionals who have never been exposed to cognitive therapy before to those who are quite experienced but wish to improve their skills of conceptualizing patients cognitively, planning treatment, employing a variety of techniques, assessing the effectiveness of their treatment, and specifying problems that arise in a therapy session.

In order to present the material as simply as possible, I have chosen one patient to use as an example throughout the book. Sally was my patient when I started writing this book several years ago. She was an ideal patient in many ways, and her treatment clearly exemplified "standard" cognitive therapy for uncomplicated, single-episode depression. To avoid confusion, Sally and all other patients mentioned in this book are designated as female, while therapists are referred to as male. These designations are made to present the material as clearly as possible and do not represent a bias. In addition, the term "patient" is used instead of "client" because that designation predominates in my medically oriented work setting.

This basic manual of cognitive therapy describes the processes of cognitive conceptualization, planning treatment, structuring sessions, and diagnosing problems which should prove useful for any patient. Although the treatment described is for a straightforward case of depression, the techniques presented also apply to patients with a wide variety of problems. References for other disorders are provided so that the reader can learn to tailor treatment appropriately.

This book could not have been written without the ground-breaking work of the father of cognitive therapy, Aaron T. Beck, who is also my father and an extraordinary scientist, theorist, practitioner, and person. The ideas presented in this book are a distillation of many years of my own clinical experience, combined with reading, supervision, and discussions with my father and others. I have learned a great deal from every supervisor, supervisee, and patient with whom I have worked. I am grateful to them all.

In addition, I would like to thank the many people who provided me with feedback as I was writing this book, especially Kevin Kuehlwein, Christine Padesky, Thomas Ellis, Donald Beal, E. Thomas Dowd, and Richard Busis. My thanks to Tina Inforzato, Helen Wells, and Barbara Cherry who prepared the manuscript, and to Rachel Teacher, B.A., and Heather Bogdanoff, B.A., who helped with the finishing touches.

CONTENTS

Chapter 1

INTRODUCTION

Cognitive therapy was developed by Aaron T. Beck at the University of Pennsylvania in the early 1960s as a structured, short-term, present-oriented psychotherapy for depression, directed toward solving current problems and modifying dysfunctional thinking and behavior (Beck, 1964). Since that time, Beck and others have successfully adapted this therapy to a surprisingly diverse set of psychiatric disorders and populations (see, e.g., Freeman & Dattilio, 1992; Freeman, Simon, Beutler, & Arkowitz, 1989; Scott, Williams, & Beck, 1989). These adaptations have changed the focus, technology, and length of treatment, but the theoretical assumptions themselves have remained constant. In a nutshell, the *cognitive model* proposes that distorted or dysfunctional thinking (which influences the patient's mood and behavior) is common to all psychological disturbances. Realistic evaluation and modification of thinking produce an improvement in mood and behavior. Enduring improvement results from modification of the patient's underlying dysfunctional beliefs.

Various forms of cognitive–behavioral therapy have been developed by other major theorists, notably Albert Ellis's rational–emotive therapy (Ellis, 1962), Donald Meichenbaum's cognitive–behavioral modification (Meichenbaum, 1977), and Arnold Lazarus's multimodal therapy (Lazarus, 1976). Important contributions have been made by many others, including Michael Mahoney (1991), and Vittorio Guidano and Giovanni Liotti (1983). Historical overviews of the field provide a rich description of how the different streams of cognitive therapy originated and grew (Arnkoff & Glass, 1992; Hollon & Beck, 1993).

Cognitive therapy as developed and refined by Aaron Beck is emphasized in this volume. It is unique in that it is a system of psychotherapy with a unified theory of personality and psychopathology supported by substantial empirical evidence. It has an operationalized therapy with a wide range of applications, also supported by empirical data, which are readily derived from the theory.

Cognitive therapy has been extensively tested since the first outcome study was published in 1977 (Rush, Beck, Kovacs, & Hollon, 1977). Controlled studies have demonstrated its efficacy in the treatment of major depressive disorder (see Dobson, 1989, for a meta-analysis), generalized anxiety disorder (Butler, Fennell, Robson, & Gelder, 1991), panic disorder (Barlow, Craske, Cerney, & Klosko, 1989; Beck, Sokol, Clark, Berchick, & Wright, 1992; Clark, Salkovskis, Hackmann, Middleton, & Gelder, 1992), social phobia (Gelernter et al., 1991; Heimberg et al., 1990), substance abuse (Woody et al., 1983), eating disorders (Agras et al., 1992; Fairburn, Jones, Peveler, Hope, & Doll, 1991; Garner et al., 1993), couples problems (Baucom, Sayers, & Scher, 1990), and inpatient depression (Bowers, 1990; Miller, Norman, Keitner, Bishop, & Dow, 1989; Thase, Bowler, & Harden, 1991).

Cognitive therapy is currently being applied around the world as the sole treatment or as an adjunctive treatment for other disorders. A few examples are obsessive–compulsive disorder (Salkovskis & Kirk, 1989), posttraumatic stress disorder (Dancu & Foa, 1992; Parrott & Howes, 1991), personality disorders (Beck et al., 1990; Layden, Newman, Freeman, & Morse, 1993; Young, 1990), recurrent depression (R. DeRubeis, personal communication, October 1993), chronic pain (Miller, 1991; Turk, Meichenbaum, & Genest, 1983), hypochondriasis (Warwick & Salkovskis, 1989), and schizophrenia (Chadwick & Lowe, 1990; Kingdon & Turkington, 1994; Perris, Ingelson, & Johnson, 1993). Cognitive therapy for populations other than psychiatric patients is being studied as well: prison inmates, school children, medical patients with a wide variety of illnesses, among many others.

Persons, Burns, and Perloff (1988) have found that cognitive therapy is effective for patients with different levels of education, income, and background. It has been adapted for working with patients at all ages, from preschool (Knell, 1993) to the elderly (Casey & Grant, 1993; Thompson, Davies, Gallagher & Krantz, 1986). Although this book focuses exclusively on individual treatment, cognitive therapy has also been modified for group therapy (Beutler et al., 1987; Freeman, Schrodt, Gilson, & Ludgate, 1993), couples problems (Baucom & Epstein, 1990; Dattilio & Padesky, 1990), and family therapy (Bedrosian & Bozicas, 1994; Epstein, Schlesinger, & Dryden, 1988).

With so many adaptations, how does cognitive therapy remain recognizable? In all forms of cognitive therapy that are derived from Beck's model, treatment is based on both a cognitive formulation of a specific disorder and its application to the conceptualization or understanding of the individual patient. The therapist seeks in a variety of ways to produce cognitive change—change in the patient's thinking and belief system—in order to bring about enduring emotional and behavioral change.

In order to describe the concepts and processes of cognitive therapy, a single case example is used throughout this book. "Sally," an 18-year-old single Caucasian female, is a nearly ideal patient in many ways and her treatment clearly exemplifies the principles of cognitive therapy. She sought treatment during her second semester of college because she had been feeling quite depressed and moderately anxious for the previous four months and was having difficulty with her daily activities. Indeed, she met criteria for a major depressive episode of moderate severity according to the fourth edition of the *Diagnostic and Statistical Manual of Mental Disorders* (DSM-IV; American Psychiatric Association, 1994). A fuller portrait of Sally is provided in the next chapter and in Appendix A.

The following transcript, excerpted from Sally's fourth therapy session, provides the flavor of a typical cognitive therapy intervention. A problem important to the patient is specified, an associated dysfunctional idea is identified and evaluated, a reasonable plan is devised, and the effectiveness of the intervention is assessed.

THERAPIST: Okay, Sally, you said you wanted to talk about a problem with finding a part-time job?

PATIENT: Yeah. I need the money . . . but, I don't know.

T: (*Noticing that the patient looks more dysphoric.*) What's going through your mind right now?

P: I won't be able to handle a job.

T: And how does that make you feel?

P: Sad. Really low.

T: So you have the thought, "I won't be able to handle a job," and that thought makes you feel sad. What's the evidence that you won't be able to work?

P: Well, I'm having trouble just getting through my classes.

T: Okay. What else?

P: I don't know. . . . I'm still so tired. It's hard to make myself even go and look for a job, much less go to work every day.

T: In a minute we'll look at that. Maybe it's actually harder for you at this point to go out and *investigate* jobs than it would be for you to go to a job that you already had. In any case, any other evidence that you couldn't handle a job, assuming that you can get one?

P: . . . No, not that I can think of.

T: Any evidence on the other side? That you *might* be able to handle a job?

P: I did work last year. And that was on top of school and other activities. But this year . . . I just don't know.

T: Any other evidence that you could handle a job?

P: I don't know. . . . It's possible I could do something that doesn't take much time. And that isn't too hard.

T: What might that be?

P: A sales job maybe. I did that last year.

T: Any ideas of where you could work?

P: Actually, maybe The [University] Bookstore. I saw a notice that they're looking for new clerks.

T: Okay. And what would be the *worst* that could happen if you did get a job at the bookstore?

P: I guess if I couldn't do it.

T: And you'd live through that?

P: Yeah, sure. I guess I'd just quit.

T: And what would be the *best* that could happen?

P: Uh . . . that I'd be able to do it easily.

T: And what's the most *realistic* outcome?

P: It probably won't be easy, especially at first. But I might be able to do it.

T: What's the effect of believing this original thought, "I won't be able to handle a job."

P: Makes me feel sad. . . . Makes me not even try.

T: And what's the effect of changing your thinking, of realizing that possibly you could work in the bookstore?

P: I'd feel better. I'd be more likely to apply for the job.

T: So what do you want to do about this?

P: Go to the bookstore. I could go this afternoon.

T: How likely are you to go?

P: Oh, I guess I will. I will go.

T: And how do you feel now?

P: A little better. A little more nervous, maybe. But a little more hopeful, I guess.

Here Sally is easily able to identify and evaluate her dysfunctional thought, "I won't be able to handle a job," with standard questions (see

Chapter 8). Many patients, faced with a similar problem, require far more therapeutic effort before they are willing to follow through behaviorally. Although therapy must be tailored to the individual, there are, nevertheless, certain principles that underlie cognitive therapy for all patients.

Principle No. 1. Cognitive therapy is based on an ever-evolving formulation of the patient and her problems in cognitive terms. Sally's therapist seeks to conceptualize her difficulties in three time frames. From the beginning, he identifies her *current thinking* that helps maintain Sally's feelings of sadness ("I'm a failure, I can't do anything right, I'll never be happy") and her *problematic behaviors* (isolating herself, spending an inordinate amount of time in bed, avoiding asking for help). Note that these problematic behaviors both flow from and in turn reinforce Sally's dysfunctional thinking. Second, he identifies *precipitating factors* that influenced Sally's perceptions at the onset of her depression (e.g., being away from home for the first time and struggling in her studies contributed to her belief that she was inadequate). Third, he hypothesizes about key *developmental events* and her *enduring patterns of interpreting* these events that may have predisposed her to depression (e.g., Sally has had a lifelong tendency to attribute personal strengths and achievement to luck but views her [relative] weaknesses as a reflection of her "true" self).

Her therapist bases his formulation on the data Sally provides at their very first meeting and continues to refine this conceptualization throughout therapy as more data are obtained. At strategic points, he shares the conceptualization with her to ensure that it "rings true" to her. Moreover, throughout therapy he helps Sally view her experience through the cognitive model. She learns, for example, to identify the thoughts associated with her distressing affect and to evaluate and formulate more adaptive responses to her thinking. Doing so improves how she feels and often leads to her behaving in a more functional way.

Principle No. 2. Cognitive therapy requires a sound therapeutic alliance. Sally, like many patients with uncomplicated depression and anxiety disorders, has little difficulty trusting and working with her therapist, who demonstrates all the basic ingredients necessary in a counseling situation: warmth, empathy, caring, genuine regard, and competence. Her therapist shows his regard for Sally by making empathic statements, listening closely and carefully, accurately summarizing her thoughts and feelings, and being realistically optimistic and upbeat. He also asks Sally for feedback at the end of each session to ensure that she feels understood and positive about the session.

Other patients, particularly those with personality disorders, require a far greater emphasis on the therapeutic relationship in order to forge a good working alliance (Beck et al., 1990; Young, 1990). Had Sally required it, her therapist would have spent more time building their alliance through various means, including having Sally periodically identify and evaluate her thoughts about him.

Principle No. 3. Cognitive therapy emphasizes collaboration and active participation. Sally's therapist encourages her to view therapy as teamwork; together they decide such things as what to work on each session, how often they should meet, and what Sally should do between sessions for therapy homework. At first, her therapist is more active in suggesting a direction for therapy sessions and in summarizing what they have discussed during a session. As Sally becomes less depressed and more socialized into therapy, her therapist encourages her to become increasingly active in the therapy session: deciding which topics to talk about, identifying the distortions in her thinking, summarizing important points, and devising homework assignments.

Principle No. 4. Cognitive therapy is goal oriented and problem focused. Sally's therapist asks her in their initial session to enumerate her problems and set specific goals. For example, an initial problem involves feeling isolated. With guidance, Sally states a goal in behavioral terms: to initiate new friendships and become more intimate with current friends. Her therapist helps her evaluate and respond to thoughts that interfere with her goal, such as, "I have nothing to offer anyone. They probably won't want to be with me." First, he helps Sally evaluate the validity of these thoughts in the office through an examination of the evidence. Then Sally is willing to test the thoughts more directly through experiments in which she initiates plans with an acquaintance and a friend. Once she recognizes and corrects the distortion in her thinking, Sally is able to benefit from straightforward problem-solving to improve her relationships.

Thus, the therapist pays particular attention to the obstacles that prevent the patient from solving problems and reaching goals herself. Many patients who functioned well before the onset of their disorder may not need direct training in problem-solving. Instead, they benefit from evaluation of dysfunctional ideas that impede their use of their previously acquired skills. Other patients are deficient in problem-solving and do need direct instruction to learn these strategies. The therapist, therefore, needs to conceptualize the individual patient's specific difficulties and assess the appropriate level of intervention.

Principle No. 5. Cognitive therapy initially emphasizes the present. The treatment of most patients involves a strong focus on current problems and on specific situations that are distressing to the patient. Resolution and/or a more realistic appraisal of situations that are currently distressing usually lead to symptom reduction. The cognitive therapist, therefore, generally tends to start therapy with an examination of here-and-now problems, regardless of diagnosis. Attention shifts to the past in three circumstances: when the patient expresses a strong predilection to do so; when work directed toward current problems produces little or no cognitive, behavioral, and emotional change; or when the therapist judges that it is important to understand how and when important dysfunctional ideas originated and how these ideas affect the patient today. Sally's therapist, for example, discusses childhood events with her midway through therapy to help her identify a set of beliefs she learned as a child: "If I achieve highly, it means I'm an okay person," and "If I don't achieve highly, it means I'm a failure." Her therapist helps her evaluate the validity of these beliefs both in the past and present. Doing so leads Sally, in part, to the development of more functional, more reasonable beliefs. If Sally had had a personality disorder, her therapist would have spent proportionally more time discussing her developmental history and childhood origin of beliefs and coping behaviors.

Principle No. 6. Cognitive therapy is educative, aims to teach the patient to be her own therapist, and emphasizes relapse prevention. In their first session, Sally's therapist educates her about the nature and course of her disorder, about the process of cognitive therapy, and about the cognitive model (i.e., how her thoughts influence her emotions and behavior). He not only helps her to set goals, identify and evaluate thoughts and beliefs, and plan behavioral change, but also teaches her *how* to do so. At each session, he encourages Sally to record in writing important ideas she has learned so she can benefit from her new understanding in the ensuing weeks and also after the end of their therapy together.

Principle No. 7. Cognitive therapy aims to be time limited. Most straightforward patients with depression and anxiety disorders are treated for 4 to 14 sessions. Sally's therapist has the same goals for her as for all his patients: to provide symptom relief, to facilitate a remission of the disorder, to help her resolve her most pressing problems, and to teach her tools so that she will more likely avoid relapse. Sally initially has weekly therapy sessions. (Had her depression been more severe or had she been suicidal, they may have arranged more frequent sessions.) After 2 months, they collaboratively decide to experiment with biweekly sessions, then with monthly sessions. Even after termination, they plan periodic "booster" sessions every 3 months for a year.

Not all patients make enough progress in just a few months, however. Some patients require 1 or 2 years of therapy (or possibly longer) to modify very rigid dysfunctional beliefs and patterns of behavior that contribute to their chronic distress.

Principle No. 8. Cognitive therapy sessions are structured. No matter what the diagnosis or stage of treatment, the cognitive therapist tends to adhere to a set structure in every session. Sally's therapist checks her mood, asks for a brief review of the week, collaboratively sets an agenda for the session, elicits feedback about the previous session, reviews homework, discusses the agenda items, sets new homework, frequently summarizes, and seeks feedback at the end of each session. This structure remains constant throughout therapy. As Sally becomes less depressed, her therapist encourages her to take more of a lead in contributing to the agenda, setting her homework assignments, and evaluating and responding to her thoughts. Following a set format makes the process of therapy more understandable for both Sally and her therapist and increases the likelihood that Sally will be able to do self-therapy after termination. This format also focuses attention on what is most important to Sally and maximizes use of therapy time.

Principle No. 9. Cognitive therapy teaches patients to identify, evaluate, and respond to their dysfunctional thoughts and beliefs. The transcript presented earlier in this chapter illustrates how Sally's therapist helps her focus on a specific problem (finding a part-time job), identify her dysfunctional thinking (by asking what was going through her mind), evaluate the validity of her thought (through examining the evidence that seems to support its accuracy and the evidence that seems to contradict it), and devise a plan of action. He does so through gentle *Socratic questioning*, which helps foster Sally's sense that he is truly interested in *collaborative empiricism*, that is, helping her determine the accuracy and utility of her ideas via a careful review of data (rather than challenging her or persuading her to adopt his viewpoint). In other sessions he uses *guided discovery*, a process in which he continues to ask Sally the meaning of her thoughts in order to uncover underlying beliefs she holds about herself, her world, and other people. Through questioning he also guides her in evaluating the validity and functionality of her beliefs.

Principle No. 10. Cognitive therapy uses a variety of techniques to change thinking, mood, and behavior. Although cognitive strategies such as Socratic questioning and guided discovery are central to cognitive therapy, techniques from other orientations (especially behavior therapy and Gestalt therapy) are also used within a cognitive framework. The therapist selects techniques based on his case formulation and his objectives in specific sessions.

These basic principles apply to all patients. Therapy does, however, vary considerably according to the individual patient, the nature of her difficulties, her goals, her ability to form a strong therapeutic bond, her motivation to change, her previous experience with therapy, and her preferences for treatment. The *emphasis* in treatment depends on the patient's particular disorder(s). Cognitive therapy for generalized anxiety disorder, for example, emphasizes the reappraisal of risk in particular situations and one's resources for dealing with threat (Beck & Emery, 1985). Treatment for panic disorder involves the testing of the patient's catastrophic misinterpretations (usually life- or sanity-threatening erroneous predictions) of bodily or mental sensations (Clark, 1989). Anorexia requires a modification of beliefs about personal worth and control (Garner & Bemis, 1985). Substance abuse treatment focuses on negative beliefs about the self and facilitating or permission granting beliefs about substance use (Beck, Wright, Newman, & Liese, 1993). Brief descriptions of these and other disorders can be found in Chapter 16.

DEVELOPING AS A COGNITIVE THERAPIST

To the untrained observer, cognitive therapy sometimes appears deceptively simple. The *cognitive model*, that one's thoughts influence one's emotions and behavior, is quite straightforward. Experienced cognitive therapists, however, accomplish many tasks at once: conceptualizing the case, building rapport, socializing and educating the patient, identifying problems, collecting data, testing hypotheses, and summarizing. The novice cognitive therapist, in contrast, usually needs to be more deliberate and structured, concentrating on one element at a time. Although the ultimate goal is to interweave the elements and conduct therapy as effectively and efficiently as possible, beginners must first master the technology of cognitive therapy, which is best done in a straightforward manner.

Developing expertise as a cognitive therapist can be viewed in three stages. (These descriptions presuppose the therapist's proficiency in demonstrating empathy, concern, and competence to patients.) In Stage 1, therapists learn to structure the session and to use basic techniques. Equally important, they learn basic skills of conceptualizing a case in cognitive terms based on an intake evaluation and data gained in session.

In Stage 2, therapists begin integrating their conceptualization with their knowledge of techniques. They strengthen their ability to understand the flow of therapy and are more easily able to identify critical goals of therapy. Therapists become more skillful at conceptualizing patients, refining their conceptualization during the therapy session itself, and using the conceptualization to make decisions about interventions. They expand their repertoire of techniques and become more proficient in selecting, timing, and implementing appropriate techniques.

Therapists at Stage 3 more automatically integrate new data into the conceptualization. They refine their ability to make hypotheses to confirm or disconfirm their view of the patient. They vary the structure and techniques of basic cognitive therapy as appropriate, particularly for difficult cases such as personality disorders.

HOW TO USE THIS BOOK

This book is intended for individuals at any stage of experience and skill development who lack mastery in the fundamental building blocks of cognitive conceptualization and treatment. It is critical to have mastered the basic elements of cognitive therapy in order to understand how and when to vary standard treatment for individual patients.

Your growth as a cognitive therapist will be enhanced if you start applying the tools described in this book to yourself. First, as you read, begin to conceptualize your own thoughts and beliefs. In the next chapter, you will learn more about the cognitive model: How you feel emotionally at a given time (and how you react physically and behaviorally) is influenced by how you perceive a situation and specifically by what is going through your mind. As of right now, start attending to your own shifts in affect. When you notice that your mood has changed or intensified in a negative direction or when you notice bodily sensations associated with negative affect, ask yourself what emotion you are experiencing, as well as the cardinal question of cognitive therapy:

> What was just going through my mind?

In this way, you will teach yourself to identify your own thoughts, specifically your "automatic thoughts," which are explained further in the next chapter. Teaching yourself the basic skills of cognitive therapy using yourself as the subject will enhance your ability to teach your patients these same skills.

It will be particularly useful to identify your automatic thoughts as you are reading this book and trying techniques with your patients. If, for instance, you find yourself feeling slightly distressed, ask yourself, "What was just going through my mind?" You may uncover automatic thoughts such as:

> "This is too hard."
> "I may not be able to master this."
> "This doesn't feel comfortable to me."
> "What if I try it and it doesn't work?"

Experienced therapists whose primary orientation has not been cognitive may be aware of a different set of automatic thoughts:

"This won't work."
"The patient won't like it."
"It's too superficial/structured/unempathetic/simple."

Having uncovered your thoughts, you can note them and refocus on your reading or turn to Chapters 8 and 9 which describe how to evaluate and respond to automatic thoughts. By turning the spotlight on your own thoughts, not only can you boost your cognitive therapy skills, but you can also take the opportunity to modify dysfunctional thoughts and influence your mood (and behavior), making you more receptive to learning.

A common analogy used for patients is also applicable to the beginning cognitive therapist. Learning the skills of cognitive therapy is similar to learning any other skill. Do you remember learning to drive or type or use a computer? At first, did you feel a little awkward? Did you have to pay a great deal of attention to small details and motions that now come smoothly and automatically to you? Did you ever feel discouraged? As you progressed, did the process make more and more sense and feel more and more comfortable? Did you finally master it to the point where you were able to perform the task with relative ease and confidence? Most people have had just such an experience learning a skill in which they are now proficient.

The process of learning is the same for the beginning cognitive therapist. As you will learn to do for your patients, keep your goals small, well defined, and realistic. Give yourself credit for small gains. Compare your progress to your level of ability before you started reading this book or to the time you first started learning about cognitive therapy. Be cognizant of opportunities to respond to negative thoughts in which you unfairly compare yourself to experienced cognitive therapists or in which you undermine your confidence by contrasting your current level of skill with your ultimate objectives.

Finally, the chapters of this book are designed to be read in the order presented. Readers might be eager to skip over introductory chapters in order to jump to the sections on techniques. You are urged, however, to attend carefully to the next chapter on conceptualization because a thorough understanding of a patient's cognitive makeup is necessary in order to choose techniques effectively. Chapters 3, 4, and 5 outline the structure of therapy sessions. Chapters 6 through 11 describe the basic building blocks of cognitive therapy: identifying and adaptively responding to automatic thoughts and beliefs. Additional cognitive and behavioral techniques are provided in Chapter 12, and imagery is discussed in Chapter 13. Chapter 14 describes homework. Chapter 15 outlines issues of termination and relapse prevention. These preceding chapters lay the groundwork for Chapters 16 and 17: planning treatment and diagnosing problems in therapy. Finally, Chapter 18 offers guidelines in progressing as a cognitive therapist.

Chapter 2

COGNITIVE CONCEPTUALIZATION

A cognitive conceptualization provides the framework for the therapist's understanding of a patient. He asks himself the following questions to initiate the process of formulating a case:

- What is the patient's diagnosis?
- What are her current problems; how did these problems develop and how are they maintained?
- What dysfunctional thoughts and beliefs are associated with the problems; what reactions (emotional, physiological, and behavioral) are associated with her thinking?

Then the therapist hypothesizes how it is that the patient developed this particular psychological disorder:

- What early learnings and experiences (and perhaps genetic predispositions) contribute to her problems today?
- What are her underlying beliefs (including attitudes, expectations, and rules) and thoughts?
- How has she coped with her dysfunctional beliefs? What cognitive, affective, and behavioral mechanisms, positive and negative, has she developed to cope with her dysfunctional beliefs? How did (and does) she view herself, others, her personal world, her future?
- What stressors contributed to her psychological problems or interfere with her ability to solve these problems?

The therapist begins to construct a cognitive conceptualization during his first contact with a patient and continues to refine his conceptualization until their last session. This organic, evolving formulation helps him to plan for efficient and effective therapy (Persons, 1989). In this chapter, the cognitive model, the theoretical basis of cognitive therapy, is described. The relationship of thoughts and beliefs is then discussed and the case example of Sally, used throughout this book, is presented.

THE COGNITIVE MODEL

Cognitive therapy is based on the *cognitive model*, which hypothesizes that people's emotions and behaviors are influenced by their perception of events. It is not a situation in and of itself that determines what people feel but rather the way in which they *construe* a situation (Beck, 1964; Ellis, 1962). Imagine, for example, a situation in which several people are reading a basic text on cognitive therapy. They have quite different emotional responses to this situation based on what is going through their minds as they read.

> Reader A thinks, "Hey, this really makes sense. Finally, a book that will really teach me to be a good therapist!" Reader A feels mildly excited.
> Reader B, on the other hand, thinks, "This stuff is too simplistic. It will never work," and feels disappointed.
> Reader C has the following thoughts: "This book isn't what I expected. What a waste of money." Reader C is disgusted.
> Reader D thinks, "I really need to learn all this. What if I don't understand it? What if I never get good at it?" and feels anxious.
> Reader E has different thoughts: "This is just too hard. I'm so dumb. I'll never master this. I'll never make it as a therapist." Reader E feels sad.

So the way people feel is associated with the way in which they interpret and think about a situation. *The situation itself does not directly determine how they feel*; their emotional response is mediated by their perception of the situation. The cognitive therapist is particularly interested in the level of thinking that operates simultaneously with the more obvious, surface level of thinking.

For example, while you are reading this text, you may notice a number of levels in your thinking. Part of your mind is focusing on the information in the text; that is, you are trying to understand and integrate some factual information. At another level, however, you may be having some quick, evaluative thoughts. These thoughts are called *automatic thoughts* and are not the result of deliberation or reasoning. Rather, these thoughts seem to spring up automatically; they are often quite rapid and brief. You may be barely aware of these thoughts; you are far more likely to be aware of the emotion that follows. As a result, you most likely uncritically accept your automatic thoughts as true. You can learn, however, to identify your automatic thoughts by attending to your shifts in affect. When you notice that you are feeling dysphoric, ask yourself: *What was going through my mind just then?*

Having identified your automatic thoughts, you can, and probably already do to some extent, evaluate the validity of your thoughts. If you find your interpretation is erroneous and you correct it, you probably discover that your mood improves. In cognitive terms, when dysfunctional thoughts are subjected to rational reflection, one's emotions generally change. Chapter 8 offers specific guidelines on how to evaluate automatic thoughts.

But where do automatic thoughts spring from? What makes one person construe a situation differently from another person? Why may the same person interpret an identical event differently at one time than at another? The answer has to do with more enduring cognitive phenomena: beliefs.

BELIEFS

Beginning in childhood, people develop certain beliefs about themselves, other people, and their worlds. Their most central or *core beliefs* are understandings that are so fundamental and deep that they often do not articulate them, even to themselves. These ideas are regarded by the person as absolute truths, just the way things "are." For example, Reader E, who thought he was too dumb to master this text, might have the core belief, "I'm incompetent." This belief may operate only when he is in a depressed state or it may be activated much of the time. When this core belief is activated, Reader E interprets situations through the lens of this belief, even though the interpretation may, on a rational basis, be patently untrue. Reader E, however, tends to focus selectively on information that confirms the core belief, disregarding or discounting information that is to the contrary. In this way he maintains the belief even though it is inaccurate and dysfunctional.

For example, Reader E did not consider that other intelligent, competent people might not fully understand the material in their first reading. Nor did he entertain the possibility that the author had not presented the material well. He did not recognize that his difficulty in comprehension could be due to a lack of concentration rather than a lack of brain power. He forgot that he often had difficulty initially when presented with a body of new information but later had an excellent track record of mastery. Because his incompetence belief was activated, he automatically interpreted the situation in a highly negative, self-critical way.

Core beliefs are the most fundamental level of belief; they are global, rigid, and overgeneralized. *Automatic thoughts*, the actual words or images that go through a person's mind, are situation specific and may be considered the most superficial level of cognition. The following section describes the class of *intermediate beliefs* that exists between the two.

ATTITUDES, RULES, AND ASSUMPTIONS

Core beliefs influence the development of an intermediate class of beliefs which consists of (often unarticulated) attitudes, rules, and assumptions. Reader E, for example, had the following intermediate beliefs:

Attitude: "It's terrible to be incompetent."
Rules/expectations: "I must work as hard as I can all the time."
Assumption: "If I work as hard as I can, I may be able to do some
    things that other people can do easily."

These beliefs influence his view of a situation, which in turn influences how he thinks, feels, and behaves. The relationship of these intermediate beliefs to core beliefs and automatic thoughts is depicted below:

Core beliefs
↓
Intermediate beliefs
(rules, attitudes, assumptions)
↓
Automatic thoughts

How do the core beliefs and intermediate beliefs arise? People try to make sense of their environment from their early developmental stages. They need to organize their experience in a coherent way in order to function adaptively (Rosen, 1988). Their interactions with the world and other people lead to certain understandings or learnings, their beliefs, which may vary in their accuracy and functionality. What is of particular significance to the cognitive therapist is that beliefs that are dysfunctional can be unlearned and new beliefs that are more reality based and functional can be developed and learned through therapy.

The usual course of treatment in cognitive therapy involves an initial emphasis on automatic thoughts, those cognitions closest to conscious awareness. The therapist teaches the patient to identify, evaluate, and modify her thoughts in order to produce symptom relief. Then the beliefs that underlie the dysfunctional thoughts and cut across many situations become the focus of treatment. Relevant intermediate-level beliefs and core beliefs are evaluated in various ways and subsequently modified so that patients' conclusions about and perceptions of events change. This deeper modification of more fundamental beliefs makes patients less likely to relapse in the future (Evans et al., 1992; Hollon, DeRubeis, & Seligman, 1992).

RELATIONSHIP OF BEHAVIOR
TO AUTOMATIC THOUGHTS

The cognitive model, as it has been explained to this point, can be illustrated as follows:

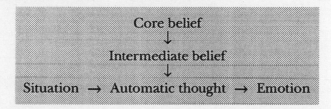

In a specific situation, one's underlying beliefs influence one's perception, which is expressed by situation-specific automatic thoughts. These thoughts, in turn, influence one's emotions.

Proceeding one step further, automatic thoughts also influence behavior and often lead to a physiological response, as illustrated in Figure 2.1.

The reader who has the thoughts, "This is too hard. I'll never understand this," feels sad, experiences a sense of heaviness in his abdomen, and closes the book. Of course, had he been able to *evaluate* his thinking, his emotions, physiology, and behavior may have been positively affected. For example, he may have responded to his thoughts by saying, "Wait a minute. This may be hard, but it's not necessarily impossible. I've been able to understand this type of book before. If I keep at it, I'll probably understand it better." Had he responded in such a way, he may have reduced his sadness and kept reading.

To summarize, this reader felt sad because of his thoughts in a particular situation. Why did he have these thoughts when another reader did not? Unarticulated core beliefs about his incompetence influenced his perception of the situation.

As explained in the beginning of this chapter, it is essential for the therapist to learn to conceptualize patients' difficulties in cognitive terms in order to determine how to proceed in therapy—when to work on a specific goal, automatic thought, belief, or behavior; what techniques to choose; and how to improve the therapeutic relationship. The basic

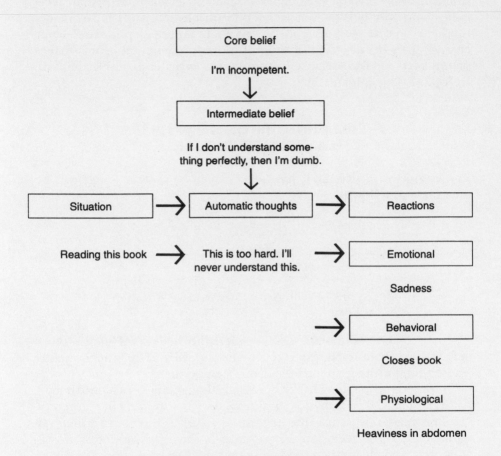

FIGURE 2.1. The cognitive model.

questions the therapist asks himself are: "How did this patient end up here? What vulnerabilities and life events (traumas, experiences, interactions) were significant? How has the patient coped with her vulnerability? What are her automatic thoughts, and what beliefs did they spring from?"

It is important for the therapist to put himself in his patient's shoes, to develop empathy for what the patient is undergoing, to understand how she is feeling, and to perceive the world through her eyes. Given her history and set of beliefs, her perceptions, thoughts, emotions, and behavior should make sense.

It is helpful for the therapist to view therapy as a journey and the conceptualization as the road map. The patient and he discuss the goals of therapy, the final destination. There are a number of ways to reach that destination; for example, by main highways or back roads. Sometimes detours change the original plan. As the therapist becomes experienced and better at conceptualization, he fills in the relevant details in the road map and his efficiency and effectiveness improve. At the beginning, however, it is reasonable to assume that he may not accomplish therapy in the most effective way. A correct cognitive conceptualization aids him in determining what the main highways are and how best to travel.

Conceptualization begins at the first contact with a patient and is refined at every subsequent contact. The therapist hypothesizes about the patient, based on the data the patient presents. Hypotheses are either confirmed, disconfirmed, or modified as new data are presented. The conceptualization, therefore, is fluid. At strategic points, the therapist directly checks his hypotheses and formulation with the patient. Generally, if the conceptualization is on target, the patient confirms that it "feels right"—she agrees that the picture the therapist presents truly resonates with her.

CASE EXAMPLE

Sally is an 18-year-old college freshman who sought therapy for persistent sadness, anxiety, and loneliness. Her intake evaluator determined that she suffered from a major depressive episode of moderate severity which had begun during the first month of school, 4 months prior to her entry into therapy.

Most questions that the intake evaluator asked Sally were fairly standard, but several were added so the evaluator and therapist could begin to form a cognitive conceptualization. For example, the evaluator asked Sally when she generally felt the worst—which situations and/or times of day. Sally replied that she felt worst at bedtime, as she lay in bed, trying to fall asleep. The evaluator then asked the key question: *"What goes through your mind at these times? What specific thoughts and/or images do you have?"*

Thus, right from the beginning, a sample of important automatic thoughts is obtained. Sally replied that she has thoughts such as the following: "I'll never be able to finish my term paper." "I'll probably flunk out of here." "I'll never be able to make anything of myself." Sally also reported an image that flashed through her mind. She saw herself, suitcase in hand, trudging aimlessly down the street, looking quite downtrodden, directionless, and desperate. During the course of therapy, Sally's therapist rounds out his conceptualization. He organizes his thinking through the use of a Case Summary Worksheet (Appendix A) and a Case Conceptualization Diagram (see Chapter 10, Figure 10.2).

Sally's Core Beliefs

As a child, Sally tried to make sense of herself, others, and her world. She learned through her own experiences, through interactions with others, through direct observation, and through others' explicit and implicit messages to her. Sally had a highly achieving older brother. As a young child, she perceived that she could not do anything as well as her brother and started to believe, although she did not put it into words, that she was inadequate and inferior. She kept comparing her performance with her brother's and invariably came up lacking. She frequently had thoughts such as, "I can't draw as well." "He rides his bike better than me." "I'll never be as good a reader as he is."

Not all children with older siblings develop these kinds of dysfunctional beliefs. But Sally's ideas were reinforced by her mother, who frequently criticized her: "You did a terrible job straightening up your room. Can't you do anything right?" "Your brother got a good report card. But you? You'll never amount to anything." Sally, like most children, placed enormous stock in her mother's words, believing that her mother was correct about nearly everything. So when her mother criticized her, implying or directly stating that Sally was incompetent, Sally believed her completely.

At school, Sally also compared herself to her peers. While she was an above-average student, she compared herself only to the best students, again coming up short. She had thoughts such as, "I'm not as good as they are." "I'll never be able to understand this stuff as well as they can." So the idea that she was inadequate and inferior kept being reinforced. She often screened out or discounted positive information that contradicted these ideas. When she got a high mark on a test, she would tell herself, "The test was easy." When she learned ballet and became one of the best dancers in the group, she thought, "I'll never be as good as my teacher." She usually made negative interpretations, which confirmed her dysfunctional beliefs. For example, when her mother yelled at her for bringing home an average report card, she thought, "Mom's right. I am stupid." She consistently interpreted negative events as demonstrating her shortcomings. In addition, when positive events such as winning an award occurred, she often discounted them: "I was just lucky. It was a fluke."

This process led to Sally's consolidating a negative core belief about herself. Sally's negative beliefs were not rock solid, however. Her father, though not around as much as Sally's mother, was generally encouraging and supportive. When he taught her to hit a baseball, for example, he would praise her efforts. "That's good . . . good swing . . . you're getting it . . . keep going." Some of Sally's teachers, too, praised her performance in school. Sally also had positive experiences with friends. She saw that if she tried hard, she could do some things better than her friends—baseball, for example. So Sally also developed a counterbalancing positive belief that she was competent in some respects.

Sally's other core beliefs about her world and about other people were, for the most part, positive and functional. She generally believed that other people were friendly, trustworthy, and accepting. And she perceived her world as being relatively safe, stable, and predictable.

Again, Sally's core beliefs about herself, others, and her world were her most basic beliefs, which she had never really articulated until she entered therapy. As a young adult, her more positive core beliefs were dominant until she became depressed, and then her highly negative core beliefs became activated.

Sally's Attitudes, Rules, and Assumptions

Somewhat more amenable to modification than her core beliefs were Sally's intermediate beliefs. These attitudes, rules, and assumptions developed in the same way as core beliefs, as Sally tried to make sense of her world, of others, and of herself. Mostly through interactions with her family and significant others, she developed the following attitudes and rules:

> "I should be great at everything I try."
> "I should always do my best."
> "It's terrible to waste your potential."

As was the case with her core beliefs, Sally had not fully articulated these intermediate beliefs. But the beliefs nevertheless influenced her thinking and guided her behavior. In high school, for example, she did not try out for the school newspaper (though it interested her) because she assumed she could not write well enough. She felt both anxious before exams, thinking that she might not do well, and guilty, thinking that she should have studied more.

When her more positive core beliefs predominated, however, she saw herself in a more positive light, although she never completely believed that she was competent and not inferior. She developed the assumption: "If I work hard, I can overcome my shortcomings and do well in school." When she became depressed, however, Sally did not really believe this assumption any longer and substituted the belief, "Because of my deficiencies, I'll never amount to anything."

Sally's Strategies

The idea of being inadequate had always been quite painful to Sally, and she developed certain behavioral strategies to shield herself from this pain. As might be gleaned from her intermediate beliefs, Sally worked hard at school and at sports. She overprepared her assignments and studied quite hard for tests. She also became hypervigilant for signs of inadequacy and redoubled her efforts if she failed to master something at school. She rarely asked others for help for fear they would recognize her inadequacy.

Sally's Automatic Thoughts

While Sally did not articulate these core beliefs and intermediate beliefs (until therapy), she was at least somewhat aware of her automatic thoughts in specific situations. In high school, for example (during which time she was not depressed), she tried out for the girls' softball and hockey teams. She made the softball team and thought, "That's great. I'll get Dad to practice batting with me." When she failed to make the hockey team, she was disappointed but not particularly self-critical.

In college, however, Sally became depressed during her freshman year. Later, when she considered playing an informal baseball game with students in her dorm, her depression influenced her thinking: "I'm no good. I probably won't even be able to hit the ball." Similarly, when she got a "C" on an English literature examination, she thought, "I'm so stupid. I'll probably fail the course. I'll never be able to make it through college."

To summarize, in her nondepressed high school years, Sally's more positive core beliefs were activated and she generally had relatively more positive (and more realistic) thoughts. In her freshman year in college, however, her negative beliefs predominated during her depression, which led her to interpret situations quite negatively and to have predominantly negative (and unrealistic) thoughts. These distorted thoughts also led her to *behave* in self-defeating ways, thereby giving her more ammunition with which to put herself down.

Sequence Leading to Sally's Depression

How is it that Sally became depressed? Certainly, her negative beliefs helped predispose her to depression. When she got to college, she had several experiences which she interpreted in a highly negative fashion. One such experience occurred the first week. She had a conversation with other freshmen in her dorm who were relating the number of advanced placement courses and exams they had taken which exempted them from several basic freshman courses. Sally, who had no advanced placement credits, began to think how superior these students were to her. In her economics class, her professor outlined the course requirements and Sally immediately thought, "I won't be able to do the research paper." She had difficulty understanding the first chapter in her statistics book and she thought, "If I can't even understand Chapter 1, how will I ever make it through the course?"

So Sally's beliefs made her vulnerable to interpreting events in a negative way. She did not question her thoughts but rather accepted them uncritically. The thoughts and beliefs themselves did not cause the depression. However, once the depression set in, these negative cognitions strongly influenced her mood. Her depression undoubtedly was *caused* by a variety of biological and psychological factors.

For example, as the weeks went on, Sally began to have more and more negative thoughts about herself and began to feel more and more discouraged and sad. She began to spend an inordinate amount of time studying, although she did not accomplish a great deal because of decreased concentration. She continued to be highly self-critical and even had negative thoughts about her depressive symptoms: "What's wrong with me? I shouldn't feel this way. Why am I so down? I'm just hopeless." She withdrew somewhat from new friends at school and stopped calling her old friends for support. She discontinued running and swimming and other activities that had previously provided her with a sense of accomplishment. Thus, she experienced a paucity of positive inputs. Eventually, her appetite decreased, her sleep became disturbed, and she became enervated and listless. Sally may indeed have had a genetic predisposition for depression; however, her perception of and behavior in the circumstances at the time undoubtedly facilitated the expression of a biological and psychological vulnerability to depression.

SUMMARY

Conceptualizing a patient in cognitive terms is crucial in order to determine the most efficient and effective course of treatment. It also aids in developing empathy, an ingredient that is critical in establishing a good working relationship with the patient. In general, the questions to ask when conceptualizing a patient are:

How is it that the patient came to develop this disorder?
What were significant life events, experiences, and interactions?
What are her most basic beliefs about herself, her world, and others?
What are her assumptions, expectations, rules, and attitudes (intermediate beliefs)?
What strategies has the patient used throughout life to cope with these negative beliefs?
Which automatic thoughts, images, and behaviors help to maintain the disorder?

How did her developing beliefs interact with life situations to make
the patient vulnerable to the disorder?
What is happening in the patient's life right now and how is the
patient perceiving it?

Again, conceptualization begins at the first contact and is an ongoing
process, always subject to modification as new data are uncovered and
previous hypotheses are confirmed or rejected. The therapist bases his
hypotheses on the data he has collected, using the most parsimonious
explanation and refraining from interpretations and inferences not
clearly based on actual data. The therapist checks out the conceptualization with the patient at strategic points to ensure that it is accurate as
well as to help the patient understand herself and her difficulties. The
ongoing process of conceptualization is emphasized throughout this
book; Chapters 10 and 11 illustrate further how historical events shape
a patient's understanding of herself and her world.

Chapter 3

STRUCTURE OF THE FIRST THERAPY SESSION

A major goal of the cognitive therapist is to make the process of therapy understandable to both therapist and patient. The therapist also seeks to do therapy as efficiently as possible. Adhering to a standard format (as well as teaching the tools of therapy to the patient) facilitates these objectives.

Most patients feel more comfortable when they know what to expect from therapy, when they clearly understand their responsibilities and the responsibilities of their therapist, and when they have a clear expectation of how therapy will proceed, both within a single session and across sessions over the course of treatment. The therapist maximizes the patient's understanding by explaining the structure of sessions and then adhering to that structure.

Experienced therapists who are unaccustomed to setting agendas and structuring sessions as described in this chapter often feel uncomfortable with this fundamental feature of cognitive therapy. Such discomfort is usually associated with negative predictions: The patient will not like it; the patient will feel controlled; it will make me miss important material; it is too rigid. Therapists are urged to test these ideas directly through implementing the structure as specified and noting the results. Therapists who initially feel awkward with a more tightly structured session often find that the process gradually becomes second nature, especially when they note the accompanying results.

The basic elements of a cognitive therapy session are a brief update (including rating of mood and a check on medication compliance, if applicable), a bridge from the previous session, setting the agenda, a review of homework, discussion of issue(s), setting new homework, and summary and feedback. Experienced cognitive therapists may deviate from this format at times, but the novice therapist is usually more effective when he follows the specified structure.

This chapter outlines and illustrates the format of the initial therapy session, whereas the next chapter focuses on the common structure for subsequent sessions. Difficulties in adhering to the structure are described in Chapter 5.

GOALS AND STRUCTURE OF THE INITIAL SESSION

Preparatory to the first session, the therapist reviews the patient's intake evaluation. A thorough diagnostic examination is essential for planning treatment effectively because the type of Axis I and Axis II disorders (according to DSM) dictates how standard cognitive therapy should be varied for the patient (see Chapter 16). Attention to the patient's presenting problems, current functioning, symptoms, and history helps the therapist to make an initial conceptualization and formulate a general therapy plan. The therapist jots down the agenda items he wishes to cover during an initial session on a therapy notes sheet (see Chapter 4, Figure 4.3).

The following are the therapist's goals for the initial session:

1. Establishing trust and rapport.
2. Socializing the patient into cognitive therapy.
3. Educating the patient about her disorder, about the cognitive model, and about the process of therapy.
4. Normalizing the patient's difficulties and instilling hope.
5. Eliciting (and correcting, if necessary) the patient's expectations for therapy.
6. Gathering additional information about the patient's difficulties.
7. Using this information to develop a goal list.

A recommended structure for the initial session encompassing these goals includes:

1. Setting the agenda (and providing a rationale for doing so).
2. Doing a mood check, including objective scores.
3. Briefly reviewing the presenting problem and obtaining an update (since evaluation).
4. Identifying problems and setting goals.
5. Educating the patient about the cognitive model.
6. Eliciting the patient's expectations for therapy.

7. Educating the patient about her disorder.
8. Setting homework.
9. Providing a summary.
10. Eliciting feedback.

If the patient is taking medication for her psychological problems, if medication is indicated, or if she is currently abusing alcohol or drugs, the therapist also adds these relevant issues to the agenda.

Before describing each session element, a caveat is in order. If the patient is hopeless and suicidal, the goals and format of the first session (or any session) are modified. It is of paramount importance to assess the patient's degree of suicidality, to discover what the patient is so hopeless about, and to undermine her hopelessness (Beck et al., 1979; Fremouw, dePerczel, & Ellis, 1990; Freeman, Pretzer, Fleming, & Simon, 1990). Crisis intervention also takes precedence above all else when the patient is in danger from others or is a potential danger to others.

It is essential to start building trust and rapport with patients in the first session. This ongoing process is easily accomplished with most patients without personality disorders. The therapist whose patient has only a straightforward Axis I diagnosis does not usually need to express his empathy through a large number of direct statements. Instead, he continuously demonstrates his commitment to and understanding of the patient through his words, tone of voice, facial expressions, and body language. Patients feel valued and understood when the therapist demonstrates empathy and accurate comprehension of their problems and ideas through his thoughtful questions and statements.

The therapist's implicit and sometimes explicit messages are that he cares about and values the patient; that he is confident they can work together; that he believes he can help her and that she can learn to help herself; that he really wants to understand what she's experiencing and what it's like "to walk in her shoes"; that he's not overwhelmed by her problems, even though *she* might be; that he has seen and helped other patients much like her; and that he believes cognitive therapy is the appropriate treatment for her and that she will get better.

As a further way of demonstrating respect for and collaboration with the patient, the therapist checks on the patient's perception of the therapeutic process and of himself as a therapist at the end of each session. Asking for explicit feedback helps strengthen the therapeutic alliance. Eliciting the patient's feedback enables the therapist to assess whether he is coming across as empathic, competent, and caring and affords him the opportunity to correct *at an early stage* any misperceptions the patient has. Patients often appreciate the rare invitation to give feedback to a professional; they receive a positive message about their partnership in therapy and ability to affect the therapeutic process. At times, a therapist and patient have a different perspective on what occurred in a therapy session; the likelihood of having the opportunity to explore these important moments is increased if the therapist consistently elicits the patient's feedback in a nonperfunctory, nondefensive manner.

SETTING THE AGENDA

As mentioned previously, an important objective in the first session is to begin to socialize the patient to cognitive therapy. As with other techniques, it is advisable first to provide the patient with a brief rationale.

THERAPIST: I'd like to start off our session by setting the agenda—deciding what we'll talk about today. We'll do this at the beginning of every session so we make sure we have time to cover the most important things. I have some items I'd like to suggest and then I'll ask you what you'd like to add. Is that okay?

PATIENT: Yeah.

T: Our first session will be a little different from future sessions, because we have a lot of ground to cover and we need to get to know each other better. First, I'd like to check on how you've been feeling. Then I'd like to hear more about what brought you to therapy, what you'd like to accomplish and what some of your problems are, and what you expect from therapy. Okay so far?

P: Uh huh.

T: I'd also like to find out what you already know about cognitive therapy, and I'll explain how our therapy will go. We'll talk about what you might try for homework, and at the end, I'll summarize what we've talked about and ask you for feedback—how you thought therapy went. . . . Is there anything you want to add to the agenda today?

P: Yes. I have some questions about my diagnosis and how long you expect I'll need to be in therapy.

T: Fine. Let me jot down your questions, and we'll make sure to get to them today. (*Jotting patient's items.*) You'll notice that I tend to write down a lot of things during our session. I want to make sure to remember what's important. . . . Okay, anything else for the agenda today?

P: No, that's all.

T: If you think of other things as we go along, just let me know.

Ideally, setting the agenda is quick and to the point. Explaining the rationale makes the process of therapy more understandable to the patient and elicits her active participation in a structured, productive way. Failure to set explicit agendas frequently results in at least some unproductive discourse as it hinders the therapist and patient from focusing on the issues that are of greatest importance to the patient. The therapist refers to agenda setting again toward the end of the session when he reviews the patient's homework. One homework assignment will be for the patient to think about (and perhaps jot down) the topic name (rather than a lengthy description) of a situation or problem she wants to put on the agenda for the next session. Most patients easily learn how to contribute to the agenda. Chapter 5 describes strategies to try when agenda setting is problematic.

MOOD CHECK

Having set the agenda in this initial session, the therapist does a brief mood check. In addition to her weekly subjective report, objective self-report questionnaires such as the Beck Depression Inventory, Beck Anxiety Inventory, and Beck Hopelessness Scale (see Appendix D) help the patient and therapist keep objective track of how the patient is doing. Careful examination of these tests can highlight for the therapist problems that the patient may not have reported verbally, for example, difficulties sleeping, decrease in sexual drive, feeling like a failure, and increased irritability.

If objective tests are unavailable, the therapist may choose to spend some time in the first session teaching the patient to provide a rating of her mood on a 0–100 scale. ("Thinking back over the past week, on the average, how has your depression [or anxiety or anger, if these are the presenting problems] been on a 0–100 scale, 0 meaning no depression at all and 100 meaning the most depressed you've ever felt?") In the transcript that follows, the therapist has finished setting the agenda and is in the process of assessing the patient's mood.

T: Okay, next. How about if we start with how you've been doing this week. Can I see the forms you filled out? (*Looks them over.*) It seems as if you're still pretty depressed and anxious; these scores haven't changed much since the evaluation. Does that seem right?

P: Yes, I guess I'm still feeling pretty much the same.

T: (*Giving rationale.*) If it's okay with you, I'd like you to come to every session a few minutes early so you can fill out these three forms. They help give me a quick idea of how you've been feeling in the past week, although I'll always want you to describe how you've been doing in your own words, too. Is that okay with you?

P: Sure.

The therapist notes the summed score of objective tests and also quickly scans individual items to determine whether the tests point out anything important for the agenda, especially noting items related to hopelessness and suicidality. He may also graph test scores or the 0–100 ratings to make the patient's progress evident to them both (see Figure 3.1).

If the patient resists filling out forms, the therapist adds this problem to the agenda so he can help her identify and evaluate her automatic thoughts about completing forms. If need be, he negotiates with the

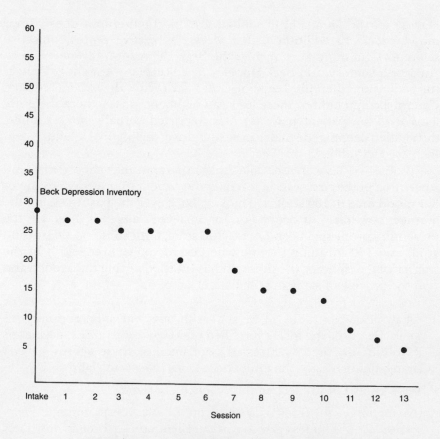

FIGURE 3.1. Graph of Sally's objective test scores.

patient, perhaps settling for 0–100 ratings or low/medium/high severity ratings in order to maintain their collaboration (see Chapter 5).

REVIEW OF PRESENTING PROBLEM, PROBLEM IDENTIFICATION, AND GOAL SETTING

In the next section, the therapist briefly reviews the patient's presenting problem. He asks the patient to bring him up-to-date, then turns their attention to identifying the patient's specific problems. As a logical extension, he then helps the patient turn these problems into goals to work on in therapy.

T: (*Summarizing first.*) Okay, we've set the agenda and checked on your mood. Now, if it's okay, I'd like to make sure I understand why you've come for therapy. I've read through the initial intake summary, and it looks as if you became pretty depressed about 4 months ago, shortly after you came to college. And you've also had a lot of anxiety, but that's not as bad as the depression. Is that right?

P: Yeah . . . I've been feeling pretty bad.

T: Anything important happen between when you were evaluated and now that I should know about?

P: No, not really. Things are pretty much the same.

T: Can you tell me specifically what problems you've been having? It helps me to hear it in your own words.

P: Oh, I don't know. Everything is such a mess. I'm doing terribly at school. I'm way behind. I feel so tired and down all the time. I feel sometimes like I should just give up.

T: Have you had any thoughts of harming yourself?

[The therapist gently probes for suicidal ideation because he will focus directly on the patient's hopelessness if the patient is actively suicidal.]

P: No, not really. I just wish all my problems would somehow go away.

T: It sounds like you're feeling overwhelmed?

P: Yes, I don't know what to do.

T: (*Helping the patient to focus and to break down the problems into a more manageable size.*) Okay, it sounds like you have two major problems right now. One is that you're not doing well at school. The other is that you feel so tired and down. Are there any others?

P: (*Shrugs her shoulders.*)

T: Well, what would you like to accomplish in therapy? How would you like your life to be different?

P: I'd like to be happier, feel better.

T: (*Getting the patient to specify in behavioral terms what "happier" and "feeling better" are for her.*) And if you were happier and feeling better, what would you be doing?

P: I'd like to be doing better in my courses and keeping up with the work ... I'd be meeting more people, maybe getting involved in some activities, like I was in high school ... I guess I wouldn't be worrying all the time. I'd have some fun and not feel so lonely.

T: (*Getting the patient to participate more actively in the goal-setting process.*) Okay, these are all good goals. How about if we have you write them on this no-carbon-required paper so we can each keep a copy.

P: All right. What should I write?

T: Here, date it at the top and write "Goal List." ... Now what was one goal? (*Guiding the patient in writing the following list with items expressed in behavioral terms.*)

> Goal List—February 1
>
> 1. Improve school work.
> 2. Decrease worrying about tests.
> 3. Meet more people.
> 4. Join school activities.

T: Okay, good. Now, how about for homework if you read through this list and see if you have any other goals to add. All right?

P: Yes.

T: Well, before we go on, let me just quickly summarize what we've done so far. We've set the agenda, reviewed your forms, talked about why you came for therapy and started a goal list.

The therapist efficiently reviews the patient's presenting problem, determines that the patient is not at risk for suicide and that there have been no significant developments since the initial intake evaluation, and helps the patient translate specific problems into goals for therapy. If the patient had been at risk for suicide, had important new information to impart, or had difficulty specifying her problems or goals, the therapist would have spent more time in this phase of the initial session (but would, of course, have had less time for other items).

Early in the session, the therapist gets the patient more actively involved by writing. He suggests to her what to write, as it is not obvious to her. (In every session, he will ask her to take notes on no-carbon-required paper [available in office supply stores] or in a notebook [from which he can photocopy] so that both he and the patient can keep a copy.) The therapist himself does the writing for patients who cannot or strongly prefer not to write themselves. Patients, including children, who are not literate can draw pictures or listen to an audiotape of the therapy session as a way of reinforcing key therapy ideas.

The therapist also guides the patient to specify a global goal ("I'd like to be happier, feel better") in behavioral terms. Rather than allowing a discussion of goals to dominate the session, he asks the patient to refine the list for homework. Finally, he summarizes what they have discussed so far in the session before moving on.

EDUCATING THE PATIENT ABOUT
THE COGNITIVE MODEL

An important overarching goal of cognitive therapy is to teach the patient to become her own cognitive therapist. Early on, the therapist elicits (and corrects, if necessary) what the patient already knows about this kind of therapy. He educates her about the cognitive model, using her own examples, and gives her a preview of therapy.

T: How about if we turn to finding out what you already know about cognitive therapy and how you expect therapy to proceed.

P: Well, I don't really know much about it, just what the counselor said.

T: What did you learn?

P: To tell you the truth, I don't really remember.

T: That's okay, we'll go over some of the ideas now. First I'd like to find out how your thinking affects how you feel. Can you think of any time in the past few days when you noticed your mood change? When you were aware that you had become particularly upset or distressed?

P: I think so.

T: Can you tell me a little about it?

P: I was having lunch with a couple of people I know and I started to feel a little nervous. They were talking about something the professor had said in our course that I didn't understand.

T: When they were talking about what the professor said, just before you began to feel nervous, do you remember what was going through your mind?

P: I was thinking that I didn't understand but I couldn't let them know it.

T: (*Using the patient's precise words.*) So you had the thoughts, "I don't understand" and "I can't let them know?"

P: Yeah.

T: And that made you feel nervous?

P: Yeah.

T: Okay, how about if we make a diagram. You just gave a good example of how your thoughts influence your emotion. (*Guides the patient in writing down the diagram in Figure 3.2 and reviews it with her.*) Is that clear to you? How you viewed this situation led to a thought which then influenced how you felt.

P: I think so.

T: Let's see if we can gather a couple more examples from the past few days. For example, how were you feeling when you were in the waiting room today, before our appointment?

P: Kind of sad.

T: And what was going through your mind at the time?

P: I don't remember exactly.

T: (*Trying to make the experience more vivid in the patient's mind.*) Can you imagine yourself back in the waiting room right now? Can you imagine sitting there? Describe the scene for me as if it's happening right now.

P: Well, I'm sitting in the chair near the door, away from the receptionist. A woman comes in, she's looking kind of smiley, and she talks to the receptionist. She's joking and looking happy and . . . normal.

T: And how are you feeling?

P: Sad.

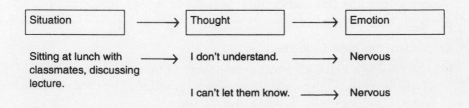

FIGURE 3.2. Sally's Session 1 notes: The cognitive model.

T: What's going through your mind?

P: She's happy. She's not depressed. I'll never be like that again.

T: (*Reinforcing the cognitive model.*) Okay. Again we have an example of how what you were thinking—"I'll never be like that again"—influenced how you felt; it made you sad. Is this clear to you?

P: Yeah. I think so.

T: Can you tell me in your own words about the connection between thoughts and feelings? (*Making sure the patient can verbalize her understanding of the cognitive model.*)

P: Well, it seems that my thoughts affect how I feel.

T: Yes, that's right. What I'd like you to do, if you agree, is to keep track this coming week of what's going through your mind when you notice your mood changing or getting worse. Okay? (*Facilitating the patient's carrying through the work of the therapy session throughout the week.*)

P: Uh huh.

T: In fact, how about if you write this assignment down [on no-carbon-required paper] so we both have a copy. "When I notice my mood changing or getting worse, ask: 'What's going through my mind?' and jot down the thoughts." Now, do you have an idea why I'd like you to jot them down?

P: I guess it's because you're saying that my thoughts make me feel bad.

T: Or they at least *contribute* to your feeling bad, yes. And to give you a preview of cognitive therapy—part of what we'll be doing together is identifying these thoughts which seem to be upsetting you. Then we'll examine those thoughts and see how *accurate* they are. Lots of times I think we'll find that these thoughts are *not* completely accurate. We should have you write down something about that, too.

P: (*Does so.*)

T: So we'll evaluate the thoughts and you'll learn to change your thinking.

P: That sounds hard.

T: Well, a lot of people think that at first, but pretty soon they find they get good at it. We'll just go step by step to teach you how to do it. But it was good that you identified your thought. Make sure if you do have any more thoughts like, "That sounds hard," to write them down so we can look at them next session. Okay?

P: Okay.

T: Do you think you'll have any trouble jotting down some thoughts?

(*Checking to see if the patient anticipates difficulties that they could problem-solve.*)

P: No. I think I'll be able to.

T: Good. But even if you can't, that's okay. You'll come back next week and we'll work on it together. All right?

P: Sure.

In this section, the therapist explains, illustrates, and records the cognitive model *with the patient's own examples*. He tries to limit his explanations to just a couple of sentences at a time and asks the patient to put into her own words what he has said so he can check on her understanding. (Had the patient's cognitive abilities been impaired or limited, the therapist might have used more concrete learning aids such as faces with various expressions to illustrate emotions.) He also makes sure that the patient writes down the most important points.

This particular patient easily grasps the cognitive model. Had she experienced difficulty in identifying her thoughts or emotions, her therapist would have weighed the benefits of using other techniques (see Chapter 6) to accomplish this objective with the possible consequence of pushing too hard (perhaps increasing the patient's dysphoria or interfering with rapport). Had he decided against further explication of the cognitive model, he would take care not to have the patient blame herself for failing to catch on. ("It's sometimes hard to figure out these thoughts. Usually they're so quick. It's no big deal. We'll come back to it another time.")

In the next section, the therapist probes for automatic thoughts in the form of visual images. Patients tend to have much more difficulty identifying these visual automatic thoughts and may not be able to provide examples. Nevertheless, they are much more likely to recognize and report images if they are alerted to them early in therapy.

T: Now, let me mention one more thing. Did you notice that I said you should ask yourself what is going through your mind when your mood changes, not "What am I thinking?" The reason I phrased it that way was because we often think in *images* or in picture form. For example, before you came in for the first time today, did you imagine what I might look like?

P: I think I had a vague picture of someone older and maybe more stern or more serious.

T: Okay, good. That picture or imagining is what we call an *image*. So when you ask yourself, "What's going through my mind?" check for both words and images. Do you want to write that down, too?

In this way, the therapist socializes the patient into recognizing that automatic thoughts may come in many different forms and even different sensory modalities, increasing the likelihood that she will be more readily aware of her automatic thoughts in *whatever* form they occur.

EXPECTATIONS FOR THERAPY

Patients often enter therapy with the notion that therapy is mystical or unfathomable and that they will not be able to comprehend the process by which they will get better. The cognitive therapist, in contrast, stresses that this kind of therapy is orderly and rational and that patients get better because they understand themselves better, solve problems, and learn tools they can apply themselves. The therapist continues to socialize the patient into therapy by imparting the message that the patient is to share responsibility for making progress in therapy. For most patients, a brief discussion, such as the one below, suffices.

T: Next I'd like to find out how you expect to get better.

P: I'm not sure what you mean.

T: Well, some patients have the idea that a therapist will cure them. Others think that they'll get better with the therapist's help but they have a sense that they are the ones who really will be doing the work.

P: I guess before I came in I thought you would somehow cure me. But from what you've said today, I guess you'll teach me things to do.

T: That's right. I'll help you learn the tools to get over the depression—and, in fact, you'll be able to use these tools for the rest of your life to help with other problems.

At the initial session, it is desirable for the therapist to give the patient a general sense of how long she should expect to remain in therapy. Usually it is best to suggest a range, $1\frac{1}{2}$ to 4 months for many patients, though some might be able to terminate sooner (or might have to, due to financial constraints or insurance limitations). Other patients, particularly those with chronic psychological difficulties or those who want to work on problems related to a personality disorder, may remain in therapy for a year or more. Most patients progress satisfactorily with weekly sessions unless they are severely depressed or anxious, suicidal, or clearly in need of more support. Toward the end of therapy, sessions may be gradually spaced further apart to give the patient more opportunity to solve problems, make decisions, and use her therapy tools independently.

The next example presents one way in which the therapist might give the patient an idea of how therapy will proceed:

T: If it's okay with you, we'll plan to meet once a week until you're feeling significantly better, then we'll move to once every 2 weeks, then maybe once every 3 or 4 weeks. We'll make these decisions about how to space out therapy together. Even when we decide to terminate, I'll recommend that you come back for a "booster" once every few months for a while. How does that sound?

P: Fine.

T: It's hard to predict now how long you should be in therapy. My best guess is somewhere around 8 to 14 sessions. If we find that you have some real long-standing problems that you want to work on, it could take longer. Again, we'll decide *together* what seems to be best. Okay?

EDUCATING THE PATIENT ABOUT HER DISORDER

Most patients want to know their general diagnosis, that they are not crazy, and that their therapist has helped others like them before and does not think they are strange. Usually it is preferable to avoid the label of a personality disorder diagnosis. Instead it is better to say something more general and jargon free, such as, "It looks as if you've been pretty depressed for the last year and you've had some long-standing problems with relationships." It is also desirable to give the patient some initial information about her disorder so she can start attributing some of her problems to her disorder and thereby decrease self-criticism.

The following transcript illustrates how to educate patients who are depressed. (It requires alteration, of course, for patients with other disorders.)

T: Now the last thing on our agenda was your diagnosis. The evaluation shows that you are significantly depressed and anxious—as are many patients we see here. I'm quite hopeful that we'll be able to help you feel better. What do you think?

P: I was afraid you'd think I was crazy.

T: Not at all, you have a fairly common illness or problem called depression, and it sounds as though you have a lot of the same problems as most of our patients here. But again, that's a good automatic thought, "You'll think I'm crazy." How do you feel now that you've found out it isn't true?

P: Relieved.

T: So correcting your thinking *did* help. If you have any more thoughts like that, would you write them down for homework so we can evaluate them at our next session?

P: Sure.

T: This kind of very negative thinking is one symptom of your depression. Depression affects how you see yourself, your world, and your future. For most people who are depressed, it's as if they're seeing themselves and their worlds through eyeglasses covered with black paint. Everything looks black and hopeless. Part of what we'll do in therapy is to scrape off the black paint and help you see things more realistically. . . . Does that analogy make sense to you?

[Using an analogy often helps the patient to see her situation in a different way.]

P: Yeah. I understand.

T: Okay, let's go over some of the other symptoms of depression that you have, too. The depression interferes with your appetite, your sleep, your sexual desire and your energy. It also affects your motivation and drive, among other things. Now most depressed people start criticizing themselves for not being the same as they had been before. Do you remember any recent times you've criticized yourself? (*Eliciting specific incidents.*)

P: Sure. Lately I've been getting out of bed late and not getting my work done and I think I'm lazy and no good.

T: Now if you had pneumonia and had trouble getting out of bed and getting everything done, would you call yourself lazy and no good?

P: No, I guess not.

T: Would it help this week if you answered back the thought, "I'm lazy"?

P: Probably. I might not feel so bad.

T: What could you remind yourself?

[Eliciting a response rather than just providing one fosters active participation and a degree of autonomy.]

P: I guess that I *am* depressed and it's harder for me to do things, just like if I had pneumonia.

T: Good. And remind yourself that as you work in therapy and your depression lifts, things will get easier. Would you be willing to write something down about this so you'll remember it this week? (*Being collaborative, yet strongly giving the message that the patient is expected to participate actively in the session and to review session content between sessions.*)

P: Yeah.

T: And here's a booklet for you to read [*Coping with Depression*; see Appendix D] that tells you more about depression.

END-OF-SESSION SUMMARY AND SETTING OF HOMEWORK

Like the capsule summaries (see p. 58) the therapist makes throughout the session, the final summary ties together the threads of the session and reinforces important points. The summary also includes a review of what the patient agreed to do for homework. In the early sessions, the therapist summarizes; as therapy progresses, the therapist encourages the *patient* to summarize.

T: Well, let me summarize what we talked about today. We set the agenda, checked your mood, set some goals, and explained how your thoughts influence your feelings. We talked about how therapy will go. We're going to be doing two major things: working on your problems and goals and changing your thinking when you find it's not accurate. Now let's see what you've written down for homework. I want to make sure you think it's manageable and that it'll help.

Homework—February 1

1. Refine goal list.
2. When my mood changes, ask myself, "What's going through my mind right now?" and jot down thoughts (and images). Remind myself that these thoughts may or may not be true.
3. Remind myself that I'm *depressed* right now, not lazy, and that's why things are hard.
4. Think about what I want to put on the agenda next week (what problem or situation) and how to name it.
5. Read booklet and therapy notes.
6. Go swimming or running three times this week.

The therapist seeks to ensure that the patient experiences success in doing therapy homework (see Chapter 14). If he senses that the patient may not carry out any part of the assignment, he offers to withdraw it. ("Do you think you'll have trouble jotting down your thoughts? [If yes,] do you think we should cross it off the list for today? It's no big deal, one way or the other.")

Occasionally a patient bristles at the term "homework." The therapist then takes care to differentiate therapy homework, which is collaboratively set and especially designed to help the patient feel better, from previous experiences (usually school homework) which involved mandatory, unpersonalized, often unhelpful assignments. Therapist and patient can also brainstorm to find a more acceptable term such as "self-help activities." Having solved the practical problem of using the term "homework," the therapist might pursue (or mentally file away for future exploration) the meaning to the patient of the word "homework" to discover whether her objection to it fits into a larger pattern (e.g., Is she sensitive to control by others? Does she feel inadequate when asked to do a task?).

A common first-session (and later-session) homework assignment involves bibliotherapy. The therapist might ask the patient to read a chapter from a layman's book on cognitive therapy (e.g., Burns, 1980, 1989; Greenberger & Padesky, 1995; Morse, Morse, & Nackoul, 1992) or an educational brochure (see Appendix D). He tries to get the patient to become actively involved in the reading ("When you read this, mark it up so you can tell me what you agree with or disagree with, what seems to fit you and what doesn't").

A second common homework assignment in early sessions is activity monitoring and/or scheduling (see Chapter 12). The goal is to get patients to resume activities in which they had previously gained a sense of accomplishment and/or pleasure.

FEEDBACK

The final element of every therapy session is feedback. By the end of the first session, most patients feel positively about the therapist and the therapy. Asking for feedback further strengthens rapport, providing the message that the therapist cares about what the patient thinks. It also gives the patient a chance to express, and the therapist to resolve, any misunderstandings. Occasionally a patient makes an idiosyncratic interpretation of something the therapist said or did. Asking the patient whether there was anything that bothered her gives her the opportunity to state and then to test her conclusions. In addition to verbal feedback, the therapist may have the patient complete a written Therapy Report (see Figure 3.3).

T: Now at the end of each session, I'm going to ask for feedback about how you felt the session went. You actually get *two* chances—telling me directly and/or writing it on a Therapy Report which you can fill out

THERAPY REPORT

1. What did you cover today that's important to you to remember?

2. How much did you feel you could trust your therapist today?

3. Was there anything that bothered you about therapy today? If so, what was it?

4. How much homework had you done for therapy today? How likely are you to do the new homework?

5. What do you want to make sure to cover at the next session?

FIGURE 3.3. Therapy report. Copyright 1995 by Judith S. Beck, Ph.D.

---

in the waiting room after our session. I'll read it over, and if there are any problems, we can put them on the agenda at our next session. Now, was there anything about this session that bothered you?

P: No, it was good.

T: Anything important that stands out?

P: I guess that maybe I can feel better by looking at what I'm thinking.

T: Good. Anything else you'd like to say or anything you'd like to put on the agenda for next session?

P: No.

T: Okay then. It was a pleasure working with you today. Would you please fill out the Therapy Report in the waiting room now and the other three forms I gave you just before our session next week? And you'll try to do the homework you wrote down on your homework sheet. Okay?

P: (*Nods*.) Okay. Thanks.

T: See you next week.

Occasionally, a patient does have a negative reaction to the first therapy session. The therapist tries to specify the problem and establish its meaning to the patient. Then he intervenes and/or marks the problem for intervention at the next session, as in the following example:

T: Now, was there anything about this session that bothered you?

P: I don't know . . . I'm not sure this therapy is for me.

T: You don't think it'll help?

P: No, not really. You see, I've got real-life problems. It's *not* just my thinking.

T: I'm glad you told me. This gives me the opportunity to say that I *do* believe that you have real-life problems. I didn't mean to imply that you don't. The problems with your boss and your neighbors and your feelings of loneliness. . . . Of course, those are all real problems; problems we'll work together to solve. I *don't* think that all we need to do is look at your thoughts. I'm sorry if I gave you that impression.

P: That's okay. . . . It's just, like . . . well, I feel so overwhelmed. I don't know what to do.

T: Are you willing to come back next week so we can work on the overwhelmed feelings together?

P: Yeah, I guess so.

T: Is the homework contributing to the overwhelmed feeling, too?

P: . . . Maybe.

T: How would you like to leave it? We could just decide now for you *not* to do homework this week and we'll do it together at our next session instead. Or you could take this sheet home and decide at home if you're feeling up to doing it.

P: I'd just feel guilty if I brought it home and didn't do it.

T: Okay, then let's plan for you not to do it. Anything else that bothered you about today's session?

Here the therapist recognizes the necessity for strengthening the therapeutic alliance. Either he missed signs of the patient's dissatisfaction during the session or the patient was adept at concealing it. Had the therapist failed to ask for feedback about the session or been less adept at dealing with the negative feedback, it is possible that the patient would not have returned for another session. The therapist's flexibility about the homework assignment helps the patient reexamine her misgivings about the appropriateness of cognitive therapy. By responding to feedback and making reasonable adjustments, the therapist demonstrates his understanding of and empathy toward the patient, which facilitates collaboration and trust.

The therapist will make sure to express at the beginning of the next session how important it is to him that they work as a team to tailor the therapy and the homework so the patient finds them helpful. The therapist also uses this difficulty as an opportunity to refine his conceptualization of the patient. In the future, he does not abandon homework altogether but ensures that it is more collaboratively set and that the patient does not feel overwhelmed.

SUMMARY

The initial therapy session has several important goals: establishing rapport; refining the conceptualization; socializing the patient to the process and structure of cognitive therapy; educating the patient about the cognitive model and about her disorder; and providing hope and some symptom relief. Developing a solid therapeutic alliance and encouraging the patient to join with the therapist to accomplish therapeutic goals are of primary importance in this session. The next chapter describes the structure of later therapy sessions and Chapter 5 deals with difficulties in structuring sessions.

Chapter 4

SESSION TWO AND BEYOND: STRUCTURE AND FORMAT

S ession two uses a format that is repeated in every subsequent session. This chapter presents the format and describes the general course of therapy from session two to near termination. The final phase of therapy is described in Chapter 15, and typical problems that arise in socializing the patient during early sessions are presented in Chapters 5 and 17.

The typical agenda for the second session and beyond is as follows:

1. Brief update and check on mood (and medication, alcohol and/or drug use, if applicable).
2. Bridge from previous session.
3. Setting the agenda.
4. Review of homework.
5. Discussion of issues on the agenda, setting new homework, and periodic summaries.
6. Final summary and feedback.

The experienced therapist may interweave the above elements to a certain extent. The beginning cognitive therapist, however, is advised to adhere to the above session structure as much as possible.

The therapist's goals during this second session are to help the patient select a problem or goal to focus on, to start solving problems, and to reinforce the cognitive model and the identification of automatic thoughts. He also aims to continue socializing the patient into cognitive therapy: following the session format, working collaboratively, providing feedback to the therapist, and starting to view her past and ongoing experience in light of the cognitive model. If the patient is feeling at all better, the therapist also starts relapse prevention work (see Chapter 15). Above all, he is concerned with building the therapeutic alliance and providing symptom relief.

BRIEF UPDATE AND MOOD (AND MEDICATION) CHECK

The mood check is usually brief and may be combined with a brief update of the week. The therapist elicits a subjective description from the patient and matches it with objective test scores. If there is a discrepancy between the test scores and the self-report, he questions the patient (e.g., "You said you've been feeling better, but your depression inventory is actually higher than last week. What do you make of that?"). He also makes a quick comparison between the objective scores of the previous session and the present objective scores (e.g., "The anxiety score is lower this week than last. *Have* you been feeling less anxious this week?"). A typical second session begins as follows:

THERAPIST: Hi, Sally. How are you feeling today?

PATIENT: A little better, I think.

T: Can I take a look at your forms? While I'm looking at them, tell me how your week went.

P: Well, okay in some ways, not so great in others.

T: What happened?

P: Well, I've been feeling a little less depressed, I think. But a lot more anxious. I've been so worried about my economics exam that I couldn't concentrate.

T: Should we put the exam on the agenda? (*Socializing the patient into briefly specifying a problem to be discussed later in the session.*)

P: Yes. And I also had a problem with my roommate.

T: Okay, I'll write that down to talk about, too. Anything else I should know about your week?

P: I guess not.

T: Okay, back to the mood check. These tests also show a small drop in depression and an increase in anxiety. Why do you think you're feeling less depressed?

P: I've been feeling a little more hopeful. I guess I think therapy might help.

T: (*Subtly reinforcing the cognitive model.*) So you had thoughts like, "Therapy might help," and those thoughts made you feel more hopeful, less depressed?

P: Yes . . . And I asked Lisa—she's in my chemistry class—to study with me. We spent a couple of hours yesterday going over some formulas. That made me feel better, too.

T: What went through your mind when you were studying with her yesterday?

P: That I liked her. That I was glad I asked her if she wanted to study together. . . . I understand it more now.

T: So we have two good examples of why you felt better this week. One, you had hopeful thoughts about therapy. And two, you *did* something different—studying with Lisa—and it sounds as if you gave yourself credit for it.

P: Yeah.

T: Can you see how in these two cases your thinking *positively* affected how you felt this week? . . . I'm glad you're feeling a little better. In a few minutes, I'll want to talk about the course of improvement, so we'll put that on the agenda, too.

Here Sally provided a brief statement about her mood. Had she started to elaborate at length, the therapist would have tried to socialize her to give a concise description (e.g., "Sally, let me interrupt you for a moment. Can you tell me in just a sentence how your depression and anxiety have been compared to the last time? . . . Or should we put 'mood check' on the agenda so we can spend more time discussing it?").

Sally also mentions two problems. Rather than initiating a discussion at this point, the therapist notes the problems for the agenda. Had he allowed her to launch into a lengthier description of the problems, he would have deprived Sally of the opportunity to reflect on what was *most* important to her to talk about during the session. He may also have had to forgo discussions of items he predicted would enable their therapy to proceed more efficiently.

Having noted a small change in her mood, the therapist asks for her explanation. If applicable, he suggests that the positive progress is a result of changes in the patient's behavior or thinking, rather than due merely to changed circumstances: "So you're feeling better but don't know why. Have you noticed any changes in your thinking this week? In the things you did?" Likewise, he seeks the patient's attribution if her mood has worsened: "Why do you think you're feeling worse this week? Could it have anything to do with your thinking or with the things you did or didn't do?" In this way, the therapist subtly reinforces the cognitive model and implies that the patient has some control over (and therefore responsibility for) her progress.

The brief mood check and review of the week create several opportunities for the therapist. He can demonstrate his concern for how the patient has been feeling in the past week. He and the patient can monitor how the patient has been progressing over the course of therapy. He can identify (and can then reinforce or modify) the patient's explanation for her progress or lack of progress. He can also reinforce the cognitive model; namely, the way the patient has been viewing situations has influenced her mood.

When reviewing objective measures, the therapist makes sure to review individual items to look for important positive or negative changes (e.g., changes in suicidal ideation or hopelessness). He might also ask for additional information not specifically covered in the tests that may be relevant to her presenting problem (number of panic attacks for panic disorder patients, number of bingeing days for bulimic patients, 0–100 rating of anger for patients with hostility problems, and so forth).

If the patient is taking medication for her psychological difficulties, the therapist briefly checks for compliance, problems, side effects, or questions. If the therapist himself is not the prescribing physician, he first obtains the patient's permission and then periodically contacts the physician to exchange information and suggestions. Although the therapist does not directly recommend changes in medication to the patient, he might help her to respond to ideas that interfere with either taking medication or reducing medication (when applicable). He might also help the patient formulate and write down specific questions about side effects, dosage, alternative medications, and so on, in order to make it more likely that the patient will seek this information from her doctor. He also suggests that while medication may be responsible *in part* for her feeling better, the patient's own efforts have probably also contributed to her improvement. If the patient is not taking medication but the therapist believes a psychopharmacological intervention is indicated, he suggests a medical or psychiatric consultation.

BRIDGE FROM PREVIOUS SESSION

The purpose of this *brief* item is to check on the patient's perception and understanding of the previous session. Knowing that she will be asked about the previous session motivates the patient to prepare for the current session by thinking about therapy during the week. If the patient does not recall her reactions or the important points from the previous session, the therapist and patient problem-solve so she can better remember the content of the current session. The therapist may suggest, for example, that the patient use the Session Bridging Worksheet (see Figure 4.1) to prepare for the next session, either mentally or in writing.

Asking for any further reactions to the past session may elicit important feedback that the patient had not previously offered. If either item appears to require more than a minute or two of discussion, the therapist may mark it down as an additional agenda item. This bridge from the last session helps to socialize the patient into the therapeutic process—giving her the message that she is responsible for reviewing the

---

SESSION BRIDGING WORKSHEET

1. What did we talk about last session that was important? What did you learn? (1–3 sentences)

2. Was there anything that bothered you about our last session? Anything you are reluctant to say?

3. What was your week like? What has your mood been like, compared to other weeks? (1–3 sentences)

4. Did anything happen this week that is important to discuss? (1–3 sentences)

5. What problems do you want to put on the agenda? (1–3 sentences)

6. What homework did you do/didn't you do? What did you learn?

FIGURE 4.1. Session bridging worksheet. Adapted with permission from Thomas Ellis, Ph.D.

content of each session and for telling the therapist whether she was bothered by anything about the therapist or the previous session.

T: Next, I'd like us to make a bridge between last session and this one, which is something we'll do at every session. First, what did you get out of the last session? What was important?

P: Well . . . a couple of things. I guess I was relieved to meet you and to hear about cognitive therapy and to know that I'm depressed and not crazy. The other thing was that how I think about something affects how I feel.

T: Good. Now a second question: Was there anything about last session that bothered you?

P: No. I thought it was good.

Had the patient brought up something that bothered her about the previous session, the therapist might have explored it with her right then or suggested that they put the problem on the agenda. Likewise, had the patient not remembered any content of significance, the therapist might have asked, "Do you remember that we talked about the connection between thoughts and feelings?" Or he might have said, "How about if we put a review of the cognitive model on the agenda?" As mentioned previously, he might also have indicated that the patient needs to take responsibility from now on for remembering important content by asking, "What could you do this coming week so you'll remember what we talked about today?" Note that a prime reason for patient's failure to recall session content is the *therapist's* failure to encourage the patient to write down the important points during the session itself.

SETTING THE AGENDA

Generally, the therapist takes more responsibility for agenda setting during early sessions and then gradually shifts responsibility to the patient. It is important for the patient to learn agenda-setting skills so she can continue with self-therapy after termination (Chapter 15).

T: Now we should set the agenda for today. We've already mentioned your exam, a problem with your roommate, and I wanted to talk about the course of improvement and some more about automatic thoughts. And, of course, I'd like to review your homework. Anything else?

P: No, I guess not.

T: This is a pretty ambitious agenda. If we run out of time, is there something we can put off 'til next week? (*Helping the patient prioritize her problems.*)

P: Ummm . . . I guess the problem with my roommate. It'll probably just blow over.

T: Okay, we'll put it last on our list and we'll try to get to it, but if not, we'll talk about it next week, if it's still relevant.

Often patients need a little encouragement initially to suggest agenda items. They may not be clearly cognizant of what has been bothering them and/or they may be unsure of what is appropriate to bring up. The therapist socializes the patient to bring up *problems* that she needs help in solving. "What problem or problems do you want to focus on today?" "What do you want to put on the agenda to get help with today?" "What should we work on today?" If there are too many agenda items, therapist and patient collaboratively prioritize items, specify the amount of time to spend on each one, and put off one or more items to the following week if necessary.

It is important to note that the therapist need not always adhere to the agenda. Indeed, under some circumstances, the therapist *should not* follow the agenda. When deviating from the agenda, however, the therapist makes such a deviation *explicit* and elicits the patient's agreement.

T: Sally, I can see that you're still really worried about your exam, but we're running out of time. Would you like to spend the rest of the session on it and postpone our other agenda items to next week? Or we could try to spend just 5 more minutes on it so we'll still have time to talk about the problem with your roommate.

P: I guess the problem with my roommate could wait until next week.

T: Okay, let me mark that in my notes and let's go back to the exam.

The therapist might suggest a change in how they spend their time during a session for a number of reasons. For example, as in the previous transcript, the patient is quite upset about a particular issue and needs more time to discuss it. Or, a new topic arises which seems especially relevant. Or the patient's mood changes (for the worse) during the session. The therapist steers the patient away from peripheral issues which were not on the original agenda and which hold little promise for helping the patient progress during the session. A notable exception occurs when the therapist deliberately (though usually briefly) engages the patient in more casual conversation to achieve a specific goal. For example, the therapist might ask about a movie the patient has just seen, or inquire about her family, or ask her opinion about current events in order to brighten her mood, facilitate their alliance, or assess her cognitive functioning or social skills.

REVIEW OF HOMEWORK

Studies suggest that patients who do homework regularly show greater improvement than do patients who do not (Persons et al., 1988; Niemeyer & Feixas, 1990). Reviewing homework at each session reinforces this behavior and communicates the value of between-session work. In our experience, if the homework is not reviewed, the patient begins to believe that it is *not* important and compliance with homework drops off dramatically. Sometimes the review of homework is relatively brief; at other times, however, it may occupy almost the entire session, especially when the issues the patient wants to discuss are contained within the homework assignment. (Homework is discussed in greater depth in Chapter 14.) Here is how a therapist might ideally review the homework:

T: Next on the agenda is the homework. What did you get done?

P: Well, I read the booklet you gave me.

T: Did you bring it with you? Could you pull it out and tell me what you learned that you think is important? (*The therapist and patient spend a few minutes discussing this.*) Anything else you have a question about? Anything else you're not clear on or you thought didn't apply to you?

P: No, that's about it. It *was* helpful.

T: Good. Now, another homework assignment was to try to catch your automatic thoughts when you noticed your mood changing.

P: I tried, but I don't think I always know what I'm thinking.

T: That's okay. We'll be talking about automatic thoughts each session 'til the end of therapy. For homework this week were you able to identify *any* automatic thoughts when your mood changed?

P: Yeah, I think so, but I didn't write them down.

T: What was the situation?

P: I was sitting in class and all of a sudden I got real anxious.

T: What was going through your mind?

P: I was thinking the exam was coming up and there's no way I'll be ready for it.

T: Good. Let me jot those down. Can we get back to these thoughts in a few minutes when we talk about the exam?

P: Yeah.

T: Any other automatic thoughts you were aware of this week?

P: Not really.

T: Okay, let's move on to your other homework assignments. Did you add anything to your goal list?

P: No. I looked at it, but I didn't think of anything else.

T: That's fine. Keep your copy, and if you do think of something else you'd like to add, let me know. And how did you do with reminding yourself that it's hard to do things because you're depressed, not lazy?

P: Pretty good. I did catch myself a few times.

The therapist intends to review all the homework assignments during the session, so he marks the automatic thoughts about the exam as a topic to pursue a little later in the session. The therapist does not have to review all the homework separately from the rest of the agenda items. Indeed, many experienced therapists integrate the homework review into a discussion of the issues on the agenda. The beginning therapist, however, needs a clear idea of where in the session he is and what is still left to be done. It is easier to adhere to the explicit structure and mark items to be discussed later. It would have been easy for this therapist, for example, to drift into a discussion of the exam and fail to review the rest of the patient's homework.

DISCUSSION OF ISSUES ON THE AGENDA, SETTING NEW HOMEWORK, AND PERIODIC SUMMARIES

Most of the time, the therapist asks the patient which agenda item she wants to start with. Doing so affords the patient the opportunity to be more active and assertive and allows her to take more responsibility. At times, the therapist takes the lead in suggesting an agenda item to start with, especially when he judges that the selection of a *particular* agenda item will result in greater progress during the session ("Is it okay with you if we start with the problem of finding a part-time job?").

The therapist interweaves his own goals as appropriate, whatever the topic under discussion. In this second session, the therapist seeks not only to help Sally do some problem-solving but also to (1) relate the topic to Sally's therapy goals, (2) reinforce the cognitive model, (3) continue teaching Sally to identify her automatic thoughts, (4) provide some symptom relief through helping Sally respond to her anxious thoughts, and (5) as always, maintain and build rapport through accurate understanding.

Agenda Item No. 1

T: Okay, let's take a look at the agenda. Where do you think we should start? We could pick a goal to work on, talk about your exam, or talk about the course of improvement.

P: My exam, I guess, I'm really worried about it.

T: Actually, that fits into two of your therapy goals, doesn't it—improving your grades and decreasing your anxiety about school.

P: Yeah.

T: Okay, can you give me an overview of what happened this week? How much did you study? What happened with your concentration?

P: Well, I meant to study all the time. But every time I sat down, I just got so nervous. Sometimes I didn't realize that my mind had wandered, and I had to keep rereading the same pages.

T: When is the exam, and how many chapters does it cover? (*Getting more data so he can help problem-solve and identify possible distortions in her thinking.*)

P: It's in 2 weeks, and I think it covers the first five chapters.

T: And how much have you read at least once?

P: About three chapters.

T: And there are still some things in the first three chapters that you don't understand?

P: A lot of things.

T: Okay. So, in a nutshell, you have an exam in 2 weeks, and you're worried that you won't understand the material well enough?

P: Right.

In this first part, the therapist just seeks a broad overview of the problem. He subtly models for the patient how to express this problem "in a nutshell." Next, he will get her to identify her automatic thoughts by having her remember a *specific* situation.

T: Can you remember a time this week when you thought about studying or tried to study and the anxiety got really bad?

P: Yes, sure. . . . Last night.

T: What time was it? Where were you?

P: It was about 7:30. I was walking to the library.

T: Can you picture it in your head now? It's 7:30, you're walking to the library. . . . What goes through your mind?

P: What if I flunk the exam? What if I flunk the course? How will I ever make it through the semester?

T: Okay, so you were able to identify your automatic thoughts. And how did these thoughts make you feel? Anxious?

P: Very.

T: Did you stop and say to yourself . . . What if I pass the exam? Maybe I'll pass the course. Maybe I'll get through the semester just fine? (*Using this problem to reinforce the cognitive model before doing problem-solving.*)

P: No.

T: What would have happened to your mood, do you suppose, if you had?

P: If I had believed it, I'd have felt better.

T: Let me tell you a little more about these automatic thoughts. We call them *automatic* because they seem just to pop into your mind. Most of the time, you're probably not even aware of them; you're probably much more aware of the anxiety or sadness they produce. Even if you *are* aware of them, you probably don't think to evaluate how correct they are. You just accept them as true. What you'll learn to do here in therapy is first to identify them and then to judge for yourself if they're completely correct or if there's some distortion in them. So, now, let's look at the first thought together. What evidence do you have that you'll flunk the exam? (*Starting the process of evaluating the automatic thought.*)

P: Well, I don't understand everything.

T: Anything else?

P: No. . . . Just that I'm running out of time.

T: Okay. Any evidence that you might *not* flunk?

P: Well, I did do okay on the first quiz.

T: Anything else?

P: I do understand the first two chapters better than the third one. The third one is the one I'm *really* having trouble with.

T: What could you do to learn the third chapter better? (*Starting problem-solving; having the patient take the lead.*)

P: I could read it again. I could look through my lecture notes.

T: Anything else?

P: (*Hesitates.*) I can't think of anything.

T: Anyone else you could ask for help?

P: Well, I suppose I could ask the teaching assistant. Or maybe the guy down the hall who took this course last year.

T: That sounds good. *Now* what do you think of your prediction that you might flunk?

P: I guess I do know some of the stuff. Maybe I *could* get help with the rest.

T: And how do you feel now?

P: A little less worried, I guess.

T: Okay, to summarize, you had a lot of automatic thoughts this week which made you feel anxious. But when you stop to evaluate these thoughts rationally, it seems likely that there are a number of things you *can* do to pass. When you really look at the evidence and answer back the thoughts, you feel better. . . . Is that right?

P: Yeah, that's true.

T: For homework this week, I'd like you to look for these automatic thoughts again when you notice your mood changing. These thoughts may have a grain of truth, but often they'll be distorted in some way. Next week we'll look for evidence together to figure out whether the thoughts you wrote down for homework are completely accurate or not. Okay?

P: Okay.

T: Now, identifying and evaluating thoughts is a skill for you to learn, like learning to drive or type. You may not be very good at it at first, but with practice you'll get better and better. And I'll be teaching you more about this in future sessions. See what you can do this week just to identify some thoughts but don't expect yourself to be good at it yet. Okay?

P: Yeah.

T: One more word about this. When you write down some thoughts this week, remind yourself again that the thoughts *may or may not be true.* Otherwise, writing them down before you've learned to evaluate them could make you feel a little worse.

P: Okay.

T: We'd better have you write some of this down now. (*The therapist repeats the assignment.*) And while we're at it, let's see if there's any homework from last week that you want to continue doing this week. And you might want to add a plan for studying for your exam. [See Figure 4.2.]

In this section, the therapist accomplishes many things at once. He addresses an agenda issue that is of concern to the patient; he ties the issue to her therapy goals; he teaches her more about automatic thoughts; he helps her identify, evaluate, and respond to a specific distressing thought; he facilitates symptom relief by decreasing the patient's anxiety; and he sets up a homework assignment and cautions the patient to have realistic expectations about learning the new skill. Chapters 6 and 8 describe in greater detail the process of teaching patients to identify and evaluate their automatic thoughts.

Agenda Item No. 2

In the next section, the therapist gives the patient some information about the course of improvement. Having just finished a segment of the session, he briefly summarizes first:

T: Okay, we just finished talking about your midterm and how your automatic thoughts really made you feel anxious and interfered with problem-solving. Next, I'd like to talk about the course of getting better, if that's okay.

P: Sure.

T: I'm glad you're feeling a little less depressed today, and I hope you continue to feel better. But probably you won't just feel a little bit better every single week until you're back to your old self. You should expect to have your ups and downs. Now I'm telling you this for a reason. Can you imagine what you might think if you expected to keep feeling better and better and then one day you felt a lot worse?

P: I'd probably think I would never get better.

---

1. When I notice my mood changing, ask myself, "What's going through my mind right now?" and jot down my automatic thoughts (which may or may not be completely true). Try to do this at least once a day.
2. If I can't figure out my automatic thoughts, jot down just the situation. Remember, learning to identify my thinking is a skill I'll get better at, like typing.
3. Ask Ron for help with Chapter 5 of econ book.
4. Read over therapy notes.
5. Continue running/swimming. Plan 3 activities with Jane [roommate].

FIGURE 4.2. Sally's homework (Session 2).

T: That's right. So I want you to remember that we predicted a possible setback, that setbacks are a normal part of getting better. Do you want to get down something in writing about that?

See Chapter 15 for a more extensive discussion of relapse prevention and a pictoral representation of the normal course of therapy.

Periodic Summaries

The therapist does two kinds of summarizing throughout the session. The first kind is a brief summary when a section of a session has been completed so both he and the patient have a clear understanding of what they have just accomplished and what they will do next.

T: Okay, so we've finished talking about the problem with your finding the time and motivation to start running again and we agreed you'd try running twice this week as an experiment. Next, is it okay if we get back to the homework you did this past week, trying to catch your automatic thoughts?

A second kind of summarizing is of the content of what the patient has presented. Here the therapist briefly summarizes the gist of the patient's statements but tries to use her specific words. Often the patient has described a problem with many details. The therapist summarizes to ensure that he has correctly identified what is most troublesome to the patient and to present it in a way that is more concise and more clear to both of them, subtly demonstrating the cognitive model over and over again. He uses the patient's own words as much as possible both to convey accurate understanding and to keep the key difficulty activated in her mind.

T: Let me make sure I understand. You were considering getting a part-time job again but then you thought, "I'll never be able to handle it," and the thought made you so sad that you folded up the newspaper and went back to bed and cried for half an hour. Is that right?

Had the therapist paraphrased the patient's ideas and failed to use her own words ("Sounds like you weren't sure if you could do well if you got a part-time job"), he might have made the automatic thought and emotion less intense and the subsequent evaluation of the thought might then have been less effective. Summaries that substitute the *therapist's* words may also lead to the patient's believing that she has not been accurately understood:

P: No, it's not that I thought I might not do well; I'm afraid I might not be able to handle it *at all*.

FINAL SUMMARY AND FEEDBACK

In contrast to the above, the therapist *refrains* from activating negative thoughts distressing to the patient in the *final summary*. Here he aims to make clear to the patient the major points covered during the session in an upbeat way. Because this is an early session, the therapist himself does the summarizing. As the patient progresses in therapy, she may take over this task. Summarizing is much more easily accomplished if during the session the patient has taken good notes that cover the most important points. The following transcript is a straightforward example of making a final summary and eliciting the patient's feedback.

T: Well, we have just a few minutes left. Let me summarize what we covered today, and then I'll ask you for your reaction to the session.

P: Okay.

T: It sounds like you've had more hopeful thoughts this week and so you've felt less depressed. Your anxiety increased, though, because you made a number of negative predictions about your exam. When we looked at the evidence that you'll flunk, though, it seems unconvincing. And you came up with several good strategies to help your studying, some of which you'll try between now and our next session. We also discussed what you should remind yourself if you have a setback. Finally, we talked about identifying and evaluating your automatic thoughts, which is a skill we'll keep practicing in therapy. Does that about cover it?

P: Yeah.

T: Anything I said today that bothered you? Anything you think I got wrong?

P: I am a little bit worried that I could have a setback.

T: Well, a setback is possible and if you do find yourself feeling significantly worse before our next session, I'd like you to call me. On the other hand, you may very well have another better week.

P: I hope so.

T: Should we put the topic "setbacks" on the agenda again next week?

P: Yes, I think so.

T: Okay, does anything else bother you or stand out about today's session?

P: No, except that I hadn't clearly realized before what I could do to help my studying.

T: Maybe we'll talk about that more next week: What ideas got in the way of your being able to do good problem-solving on your own. Okay? See you next week.

If the therapist senses that the patient has not fully expressed her feedback about the session, or if he judges that the patient may leave the session without adequate reflection about what she learned, he may ask her to complete a therapy report (see Figure 3.3), either mentally or in writing.

SESSION THREE AND BEYOND

Therapy sessions subsequent to the second session maintain the same format. The content varies according to the patient's problems and goals and the therapist's goals. In this section, the flow of therapy across sessions will be outlined. A more detailed description of treatment planning can be found in Chapter 16.

As mentioned previously, the therapist initially takes the lead in suggesting agenda items, helping the patient to identify and modify automatic thoughts, devising homework assignments, and summarizing the session. As therapy progresses, there is a gradual shift in responsibility. Toward the end of therapy, the patient herself names most of the agenda topics, uses tools such as a Dysfunctional Thought Record (see Chapter 9) to evaluate her thinking, devises her own homework assignments, and summarizes the therapy session.

Another gradual shift is from an emphasis on automatic thoughts to a focus on both automatic thoughts and underlying beliefs (see Chapters 10 and 11). Shifts in the relative emphasis on behavior changes, too, though in a less predictable fashion. Depressed patients are encouraged from the beginning to schedule activities and become more active (see Chapter 12). (A severely depressed patient may be unable to concentrate on cognitive tasks and the therapist focuses on activating her behaviorally until her depression lifts sufficiently to allow her to do cognitive work.) The therapist returns to an emphasis on behavioral change in order to have the patient test certain thoughts or beliefs or practice new skills such as assertiveness (see Chapter 12). As therapy moves into the final phase, there is yet another shift: preparing the patient for termination and relapse prevention (see Chapter 15).

The therapist keeps in mind the stage of therapy when planning an individual session. As mentioned in Chapter 2, he continues to use his conceptualization of the patient to guide therapy. The therapist jots down agenda items on the therapy notes sheet (see Figure 4.3) before a session and is prepared to eliminate his items if necessary. As the patient reports on her mood, briefly reviews the week, and specifies agenda topics, the therapist formulates in his own mind a specific goal or goals

THERAPY NOTES

Patient's name: _Sally_   **Date:** _3/15_   **Session no.:** _7_

Objective scores: _Beck Depression Inventory = 18, Beck Anxiety Inventory = 7, Hopelessness Scale = 9_

Patient's agenda:

Problem with English paper

Therapist's objectives:

Continue to modify perfectionist thinking.

Decrease anxiety and avoidance around participating in class.

Session highlights:

1. _Feeling less depressed and anxious this week._

2. _(Situation/problem)   (Automatic thought)   (Emotion)_

   English paper due tomorrow → It's not good enough → Anxious

   Intervention—Dysfunctional Thought Record—attached

   Outcome—Anxiety ↓ (reduced)

3. _Old belief:_   _If I don't get an A, it means I don't have what it takes to be a success._
   90% **(strength of belief)**

   Intervention: _Advice to Donna_ **(friend)**

   Outcome: 80% **(rerating strength of belief)**

   Intervention #2:   _Rational—emotional role-play_

   Outcome: 60% **(rerating strength of belief)**

   New belief: _I don't need all A's to succeed now or in the future._ 80%

4. _Coping card about asking questions after class (attached)._

Homework: (If patient has written homework assignment on no-carbon-required paper, just attach it without rewriting here)

DTR and credit list.

Read therapy notes and think about old and new beliefs about success.

Read coping cards 3 times a day and as needed; then ask 1 or 2 questions after class.

Spend one more hour to polish English paper.

Next session or future sessions:

See how perfectionism affects other parts of life.

FIGURE 4.3. Therapy notes.

for the session. For example, in session three, the therapist's goals are to begin teaching Sally in a structured way to evaluate her automatic thoughts and to continue to schedule pleasurable activities. In session four, he aims to help her do some problem-solving about finding a part-time job and continue to respond to her dysfunctional thoughts. He continually seeks to integrate his goals with Sally's agenda items. Thus he teaches her problem-solving and cognitive restructuring skills in the context of situations she brings to therapy. This combination of solving problems and helping patients respond to their thoughts generally allows the therapist and patient sufficient time to discuss in depth only one or two problematic situations from the agenda during a given therapy session.

In order to refine his conceptualization, to keep track of what is being covered in a therapy session, and to plan future sessions, the therapist takes notes during the session (see Figure 4.3) and keeps a copy of notes the patient takes as well. It is useful for the therapist to note the problem(s) discussed, dysfunctional thoughts and beliefs (written verbatim) and the degree to which the patient initially believed them, the interventions made in session, the relative success of these interventions, the new restructured thoughts and beliefs and the degree of belief in them, the assigned homework, and topics for the agendas of subsequent sessions. Even experienced therapists have difficulty remembering all these important items without written notes.

This chapter outlined the structure and format of a typical early therapy session and briefly described therapy across sessions. The following chapter discusses problems in following the prescribed format, while Chapter 16 describes in detail how to plan treatment before individual sessions, within sessions, and across sessions.

Chapter 5

PROBLEMS WITH STRUCTURING THE THERAPY SESSION

Problems invariably arise in structuring a session. When the therapist becomes aware of a problem, he first specifies it, then conceptualizes why the problem arose, and finally devises a solution that does not disturb the therapeutic alliance.

A common difficulty in maintaining the prescribed structure is the therapist's failure to socialize the patient adequately. The therapist may simply need to sharpen his skills at socialization, or he may need to evaluate and test his own automatic thoughts about structuring.

It is important for the therapist to realize that a patient new to cognitive therapy does not know in advance that her therapist would like her to report on the week, describe her mood, and set the agenda in a succinct way. She does not know that she will be expected to summarize a session, provide feedback, remember session content, and consistently do daily homework. In addition, the cognitive therapist is essentially teaching the patient not only certain skills but also a new way of relating to a therapist (for those who have been in another type of therapy) or a new way of relating to her difficulties so that she can adopt a more objective, problem-solving orientation.

Therefore, the therapist must often repeatedly describe, provide a rationale, and monitor with gentle, corrective feedback each of the session elements. Failure to do so usually results in the patient providing less useful information and in inefficiency in the session.

A second common difficulty involves the patient's unwillingness to conform to the prescribed structure because of her perceptions of and dysfunctional beliefs about herself, the therapist, and/or therapy. In this case, the therapist conceptualizes why the problem arose and devises a solution. At one extreme he may acknowledge the patient's discomfort but encourage her to comply as an experiment. At the other extreme, he may allow the patient to dominate and control the flow of the session—initially. With most patients, however, the therapist negotiates a compromise satisfactory to both and tries, over time, to move the patient toward the standard structure.

How does the therapist determine whether the difficulty in adherence to session structure is due to faulty socialization or reluctance in complying? He first intervenes by further socializing the patient to the cognitive therapy model and by monitoring her verbal and nonverbal responses. If it is simply a problem in socialization, the patient's response is fairly neutral (or perhaps slightly self-critical) and subsequent compliance is good. If the patient reacts negatively, she has undoubtedly perceived the therapist's request in a negative way and the therapist should elicit and explore her reaction.

A third common difficulty in maintaining the session structure arises because the therapist has imposed the structure in too controlling or demanding a fashion. The therapist diagnoses this problem through review of a tape (audio or video) of the session and remedies it at the next session: "I think I came across too heavy-handed last week. I'm sorry, I do want to make sure that you agree with how the session goes."

Typical problems with each stage of the therapy session, excluding significant mistakes by the therapist, are presented below.

BRIEF UPDATE

A common difficulty is that the patient begins the session with too detailed an account of or unfocused rambling about her week. After several such sentences, the therapist gently jumps in, relating the importance of focusing on specific problems in therapy.

THERAPIST: Let me interrupt you for a moment. It's important to me to understand the big picture of your week and to get the details later in the session. For right now, could you just tell me about your week in two or three or four sentences? Was it generally a good week? A bad week? Or did it have its ups and downs? What important things happened?

If the patient continues to offer details instead of the broader picture, the therapist might demonstrate what he is looking for.

T: It sounds to me like you're saying, "I had a pretty hard week. I had a fight with a friend, and I was really anxious about going out, and I had trouble concentrating on my work." That's the big picture I was talking about that helps me get a sense of what's really important to put on the agenda and find out more about later. Is it clearer to you now what I'm looking for when you give me an update at the beginning of the session? Is doing it that way okay with you?

The therapist might suggest later in the session that the patient mentally prepare a broad review of her week in just a few sentences before the next session.

Some patients do understand and are capable of providing a concise review but do not *choose* to do so. If the therapist has data to suggest that questioning the patient about her reluctance to comply could damage their alliance, he may initially allow her to control the update portion of the session. (Such data might include the patient's verbal and/or non-verbal reactions to the therapist's prior attempts at structuring, her direct statements of strong preferences in the therapeutic process, or her reports of a strong reaction in the past when she has perceived others as controlling or dominating.)

Extreme reactions to structuring are not common, however. The therapist can usually calmly explore reasons for the patient's reluctance and then problem-solve with her. After asking the patient to review her week more concisely and noting a negative shift in affect, the therapist might ask, "When I just asked you to give me the big picture, what went through your mind?" Having identified the patient's automatic thoughts, the therapist might then (1) help her evaluate the validity of the thoughts, (2) use the downward arrow technique (see pp. 145–146) to uncover the meaning of the thoughts, and/or (3) make an empathic statement and move straight to problem-solving, as below:

T: I'm sorry you felt I cut you off again. I can see you have a lot on your mind, and I *would* like to hear it. Would you like to continue with the update now, or should we put "update of week" on the agenda and devote a good chunk of time to it after we've checked your mood and decided what other topics you also want to put on the agenda?

This latter choice is usually better than helping the patient evaluate her thoughts at the moment if she is particularly annoyed. By expressing his concern and willingness to compromise, the therapist often modifies the patient's perception (accurate or not) that he is being too controlling.

MOOD CHECK

Common problems involve the patient's failure to fill out forms, annoyance with forms, or difficulty in subjectively expressing (in a concise manner) her general mood during the week. If the difficulty is simply faulty socialization relating to completing the forms, the therapist asks the patient whether she remembers and agrees with the rationale for filling them out and determines whether there's a practical difficulty that needs to be resolved (e.g., insufficient time, forgetting, or problem in literacy).

If the patient is annoyed at the request to fill out the forms, the therapist may ask for her automatic thoughts when thinking about or actually filling them out. If her automatic thoughts are not easily accessible, he asks for the significance of the situation to her: "What does it *mean* to you to be asked to fill out these forms?" The therapist can empathically respond to the patient's concern, help her evaluate relevant thoughts and beliefs, and/or do problem-solving. These responses are provided in the three examples below.

PATIENT: These forms are a waste of time. Half of the questions are irrelevant.

T: Yes, I understand the forms *seem* to be a waste of time to you because not all the questions apply. However, they do save a lot of time in session because I can look at them quickly and get the overall picture and not bother you with dozens of questions myself. Would you be willing to fill them out again next week and we can talk more about them then if they still bother you?

In the next example, the patient clearly expresses her annoyance through her choice of words, tone of voice, and body language.

P: These forms are a waste of time. Half the questions are irrelevant.

T: What does it mean to you to be asked to fill out these forms?

P: I'm busy. I have a lot to do. If my life fills up with meaningless tasks, I'll never get anything done.

T: I can see you feel pretty irritated. How long does it take to fill out these forms?

P: . . . I don't know. Ten minutes, maybe.

T: I know you see the forms as irrelevant, but actually they save us time in the therapy session because I don't have to ask you lots of questions myself. Could we try to problem-solve and see where you could fit in the 10 minutes a week you need to fill them out?

P: It's not that big a deal. I'll do them. I guess I'll just have to make sure to leave work a little earlier next time.

Here the therapist has the patient identify the meaning of the situation. The patient catastrophizes about the time it takes until the therapist helps her see how brief the forms actually are. The therapist does not *directly* evaluate the accuracy of the patient's ideas here because the patient is annoyed and he senses that she will perceive such questioning in a negative way.

In a third case, the therapist judges that further persuasion to fill out forms will negatively affect a tenuous therapeutic alliance.

P: (*In an angry voice.*) I hate these forms. They don't apply to me. I know *you* want me to fill them out, but I'm telling you, they're worthless.

T: I'm willing for you to skip them, or to fill them out just once in a while. I *would* like to get some clear idea of how you've been feeling during the week, though. Would you be willing to tell me verbally how angry, sad, and anxious you've been feeling on a 0–100 scale?

A different problem involves the patient's difficulty in subjectively expressing her mood, either because she does not do so concisely or because she has difficulty labeling her moods. The therapist might gently interrupt her and either ask specific questions or demonstrate to her how to respond.

T: Can I interrupt for a moment? Can you tell me in just a sentence how your mood has been this week as compared to last week? I *do* want to hear more about the problem with your brother in a few minutes, but first I just need to know whether you've generally felt better, worse, or the same compared to last week.

P: A little worse, I think.

T: More anxious? More sad? More angry?

P: Maybe a little more anxious. About the same amount of sad. Not angry really.

If the patient has difficulty labeling her mood, the therapist might respond differently:

T: It sounds like it's hard to pin down how you've been feeling. Maybe we should put on the agenda "identifying feelings."

During the session, the therapist might use the techniques described in Chapter 7 to teach the patient to specify her mood.

BRIDGE FROM PREVIOUS SESSION

Problems that arise here usually involve the patient's difficulty in remembering session content or her reluctance to express negative feedback to the therapist. One solution is to ask the patient to complete a Session Bridging Worksheet (see Chapter 4, Figure 4.1) before each session. Note, though, that difficulty in relating the most important points of the previous session is most often due to the therapist's neglecting to encourage the patient to write down these points during the session itself or to the patient's failure to follow through with a homework assignment to read her notes daily.

Difficulty in having the patient honestly express her reaction to the previous session can be handled in several ways. First the therapist can use additional encouragement, as in the example below, if he suspects the patient did have a negative reaction.

T: So you thought last session went okay. If you had been bothered by something, do you think you would have told me?

P: I think so.

T: Good, because I *do* want to tailor this therapy to you, and if there was something that bothered you, I'd really like to hear about it so we could problem-solve.

Second, the therapist could uncover the *meaning* to the patient of providing negative feedback.

T: Okay, so you were basically satisfied with our session last week. I wonder, though, would it mean something to you if you *had* been dissatisfied and told me so?

P: Oh, I wouldn't ever criticize you. I know you're doing what's best.

T: Well, thank you, but I'm only human, and I know I do make mistakes at times. What would it mean if you *did* criticize me?

P: Oh . . . I'd really be ungrateful.

T: Hmmm. I wonder if that automatically follows—that giving me feedback that I am asking for and really want means you're ungrateful. Could we put this on the agenda to talk more about?

SETTING THE AGENDA

Typical difficulties here are that the patient fails to contribute to the agenda, rambles when setting the agenda, or is hopeless about discussing problems on the agenda. The patient who fails to contribute to the agenda either is inadequately socialized or puts a special negative *meaning* on contributing. These two cases are illustrated below.

T: What would you like to put on the agenda?

P: . . . Nothing, really.

T: What problems came up for you this past week? Or, what problems do you expect might come up this week?

P: I don't know. Things are okay, I guess.

T: Then how about if we put on the agenda to look at how you're doing in terms of the goals we set at the beginning of therapy?

P: Okay.

T: And if it's all right, I'd like you to write down for a homework assignment this coming week to think about what you'd like to put on the agenda next week.

If the patient fails to set an agenda topic the following week, even in the face of an update that suggests she did experience some difficulties, the therapist might elicit her automatic thoughts about and/or the meaning of his request.

T: Did you remember to think of an agenda topic?

P: Yeah. But I don't know. I just didn't come up with anything.

T: What went through your mind as you were trying to think of a topic?

P: I don't know . . . that *you* were the doctor; you know better than I do what we should talk about.

T: How does it make you feel when I push you to think about a topic?

P: It's okay.

T: A little annoyed, maybe?

P: A little.

The therapist can then elicit the patient's expectations for therapy and help her examine advantages and disadvantages for holding these expectations.

Patients who launch into a detailed account of a problem instead of just naming the problem during agenda setting usually just require further instruction.

T: (*Gently interrupting.*) I can tell that this is an important problem. Can you just tell me the *name* of the topic right now, and we'll get back to it in a few minutes? Would you call it "a problem with my boss"?

P: Yes.

T: Good. Can you tell me the name of any other problem you'd like to put on the agenda?

A patient who persists in the next session in reciting rather than naming during agenda setting can be asked to jot down her agenda topics for homework.

A third problem in agenda setting arises when the patient feels hopeless about discussing her problems. Here the therapist tries to get her into a problem-solving mode.

T: Okay. So on the agenda so far, we've got the problems of tiredness and organizing your finances for tax purposes. Anything else?

P: (*Sighs.*) No. . . . Yes. . . . I don't know. . . . I'm so overwhelmed. I don't think any of this is going to help.

T: You don't think talking about your problems in here will help?

P: No. What's the use? I mean, you can't fix the fact that I owe too much money and I'm so tired I can't even get out of bed most mornings—not to mention the fact that I'm so far behind in my course work that I'll probably flunk out.

T: Well, it's true that we can't fix everything at once. And you do have real problems that we need to work on together. Now if we just have time to work on one thing today, which do you think will help more than the others?

P: I don't know. . . . The tiredness, maybe. If I could get out of bed, maybe I could get more done.

In this case, the therapist gives the patient the message that her problems are real, that they can be worked on one by one, and that she need not work on them alone. Asking her to make a forced choice *does* help her focus on selecting a problem and seems to help her get oriented toward problem-solving. Had the patient refused to make a choice, the therapist might have tried a different tactic.

T: It sounds like you're feeling pretty hopeless. I don't know for sure that working together we can make a difference, but I'd like to try. Would you be willing to try? Could we talk about the tiredness for 10 or 15 minutes and see what happens?

Acknowledging the patient's hopelessness and the therapist's inability to guarantee success may make the patient willing to experiment with problem-solving for a few minutes.

REVIEW OF HOMEWORK

A typical problem is that the therapist, in his haste to get to the patient's agenda issues, fails to ask the patient about the homework she did over the past week. The therapist is more likely to remember to ask about homework if he keeps before him the six elements of the therapy session (see Chapter 4, p. 45) and the previous week's therapy notes containing the written assignment. The opposite problem sometimes arises when the therapist reviews homework (unrelated to the patient's distress that day) in too much detail before turning to the patient's agenda topic. Other homework problems are discussed in detail in Chapter 14.

DISCUSSION OF AGENDA ITEMS

Typical problems here include hopelessness, unfocused or tangential discussion, inefficient pacing, and a failure to make a therapeutic intervention. *Unfocused discussion* usually results when the therapist fails to structure the discussion appropriately through gentle interruptions (guiding the patient back to the issue at hand); when he fails to emphasize *key* automatic thoughts, emotions, beliefs, and behavior; and when he fails to summarize frequently. In the following transcript, the therapist summarizes several minutes of the patient's description in just a few words and redirects the patient to identify her automatic thoughts.

T: Let me just make sure I understand. You had a fight with your sister yesterday. This reminded you of previous fights and you began to get more and more angry. Last night, you called her again, and she began to criticize you for not helping out with your mother. What went through your mind as she said, "You're the black sheep of the family"?

Pacing is often a problem for the novice therapist who overestimates how many issues can be discussed during one therapy session. It is preferable to prioritize and then to specify just one or two issues to be discussed during a session. The therapist and patient together should keep track of the time during the session and collaboratively decide what to do if time is running short. (In practical terms, this means having one or more clocks placed so both can monitor the passage of time.)

T: We only have 10 minutes left before we have to start closing down the session. Would you like to continue talking about this problem with your neighbor or finish up in the next minute or 2 so we have time to discuss the other problem with your coworker?

A third problem with discussion of issues is the *therapist's failure to make a therapeutic intervention*. Much of the time, merely describing a problem or identifying dysfunctional thoughts or beliefs related to the problem will *not* result in the patient's feeling better. The therapist should be conscious of his goal to help the patient (during the session itself) respond to her dysfunctional cognitions, solve or partially solve a problem, or set up a homework assignment designed to ameliorate the problem or help her feel less distressed.

SETTING NEW HOMEWORK

Patients are less likely to do homework when the therapist (1) suggests an assignment that is too difficult or is unrelated to the patient's concerns; (2) fails to provide a good rationale; (3) forgets to review homework assigned during previous sessions; (4) does not stress the importance of daily homework in general and of specific assignments in particular; (5) does not explicitly teach the patient how to do the assignment; (6) does not start the assignment in session, do covert rehearsal (Chapter 14, pp. 257–259), or ask standard questions about potential obstacles that might get in the way; (7) does not have the patient write the homework assignment down; or (8) noncollaboratively sets a homework assignment that the patient does not want to do.

If none of the above is true, the therapist tries to ascertain whether the patient holds dysfunctional beliefs about homework (e.g., "I should feel better without working hard"; "My therapist should cure me without my having to change things"; "I'm too incompetent to do homework"; "Homework is trivial and won't get me better"). The therapist then helps the patient specify and test her dysfunctional ideas about homework. Homework is discussed more extensively in Chapter 14.

FINAL SUMMARY

The therapist summarizes periodically throughout the session to make sure he understands what the patient has been expressing. If he has asked the patient to record important points in writing during the session, the end summary can consist of a quick review of these notes and a verbal summary of any other topics which were discussed. Failure to have the patient take notes usually leads to greater difficulty in summarizing the session and in having the patient remember the session in the ensuing week.

FEEDBACK

Problems arise when the patient is distressed at the end of a session without sufficient time to resolve the distress or when the patient fails to express her negative reaction at all. A practical solution to avoid running out of time is to start closing down the session 10 minutes before the end. Then the therapist can more effectively assign new homework, summarize the session, and elicit and respond to feedback. A sample response to negative feedback follows:

T: Anything I said today that bothered you?

P: I don't think you realize how hard it is for me to get things done. I have so many responsibilities and so many problems. It's easy for *you* to say I should just concentrate on my work and forget all about what's happening with my boss.

T: Oh, I'm sorry if you got that impression. What I *meant* to get across was that I realize you are very distressed by the problem with your boss, and I wish we could resolve that problem this week. I'd like to talk more about it next week. But meanwhile, was there something I said or did that made you think I was suggesting that you just forget all about the problem with your boss?

[The therapist next clarifies the misunderstanding.]

PROBLEMS ARISING FROM THE THERAPIST'S COGNITIONS

The problems presented above presuppose that the therapist agrees with the standard structure of the therapy session and feels competent to implement it. Below are typical therapists' thoughts and beliefs which can interfere with implementing the standard structure.

Automatic thoughts
"I can't structure the session."
"[My patient] won't like the structure."
"She can't express herself succinctly."
"I shouldn't interrupt her."
"She'll get mad if I'm too directive." *(cont.)*

> "She won't do homework."
> "She'll feel denigrated if I evaluate her thinking."

It is important for the therapist to monitor his own level of discomfort and identify his own automatic thoughts during and between sessions. He can then identify a problem, evaluate and respond to his thoughts, and problem-solve to make it easier for him to experiment with implementing the standard structure at the next session.

Chapter 6

IDENTIFYING AUTOMATIC THOUGHTS

The cognitive model states that the interpretation of a situation (rather than the situation itself), often expressed in automatic thoughts, influences one's subsequent emotion, behavior, and physiological response. Of course, certain events are almost universally upsetting: a personal assault, rejection, or failure. People with psychological disorders, however, often misconstrue neutral or even positive situations and thus their automatic thoughts are biased. By critically examining their thoughts and correcting thinking errors, they often feel better.

This chapter describes the characteristics of automatic thoughts along with techniques to identify patients' automatic thoughts, explain automatic thoughts to patients, differentiate between automatic thoughts and interpretations, and teach patients to identify their own automatic thoughts. The next chapter focuses on negative emotions: how to teach patients to differentiate automatic thoughts from emotions and to identify and rate the intensity of emotions.

CHARACTERISTICS OF AUTOMATIC THOUGHTS

Automatic thoughts are a stream of thinking that coexists with a more manifest stream of thought (Beck, 1964). These thoughts are not peculiar to people with psychological distress; they are an experience common to us all. Most of the time we are barely aware of these thoughts, though with just a little training we can easily bring these thoughts into consciousness. When we become aware of our thoughts, we may automatically do a reality check if we are not suffering from psychological dysfunction.

A reader of this text, for example, while focusing on the content of this chapter, may have the automatic thought, "I don't understand this," and feel slightly anxious. He may, however, spontaneously (i.e., without conscious awareness) respond to the thought in a productive way: "I *do* understand *some* of it; let me just reread this section again."

This kind of automatic reality testing and responding to negative thoughts is a common experience. People who are in distress, however, may not engage in this kind of critical examination. Cognitive therapy teaches them tools to evaluate their thoughts in a conscious, structured way, especially when they are upset.

Sally, for example, when she is reading an economics chapter, has the same thought as the reader above. "I don't understand this." Her thinking becomes even more extreme, however: "And I'll *never* understand it." She accepts these thoughts as correct and feels quite sad. After learning tools of cognitive therapy, however, she is able to use her negative emotion as a cue to look for, identify, and evaluate her thoughts and thereby develop a more adaptive response: "Wait a minute, it's not necessarily true that I'll never understand this. I am having some trouble now. But if I reread it or come back to it when I'm fresher, I may understand it more. Anyway, understanding it isn't crucial to my survival, and I can ask someone else to explain it to me if need be."

Although automatic thoughts seem to pop up spontaneously, they become fairly predictable once the patient's underlying beliefs are identified. The cognitive therapist is concerned with identifying those thoughts that are dysfunctional, that is, those that distort reality, that are emotionally distressing and/or interfere with the patient's ability to reach her goals. Dysfunctional automatic thoughts are almost always negative unless the patient is manic or hypomanic, has a narcissistic personality disorder, or is a substance abuser.

Automatic thoughts are usually quite brief, and the patient is often more aware of the *emotion* she feels as a result of the thought than of the thought itself. Sitting in session, for example, a patient may be somewhat aware of feeling anxious, sad, irritated, or embarrassed but unaware of her automatic thoughts until her therapist questions her.

The emotion the patient feels is logically connected to the content of the automatic thought. For example, Sally thinks, "I'm such a dope. I don't really understand what [my therapist] is saying," and feels sad. Another time she thinks, "He's watching the clock. I'm just another case to him," and feels slightly angry. When she has the thoughts, "What if this therapy doesn't work? What will I do next?" Sally feels anxious.

Automatic thoughts are often in "shorthand" form but can be easily spelled out when the therapist asks for the *meaning* of the thought. For example, "Oh, no!" may be translated as "[My therapist] is going to give me too much homework." "Damn!" may be the expression of an idea such as "I left my appointment book at home and I can't schedule another appointment with my therapist today; I'm so stupid."

Automatic thoughts may be in verbal form, visual form (images), or both. In addition to her verbal automatic thought ("Oh, no!") Sally had an image of herself, alone at her desk late at night, toiling over her therapy homework (see Chapter 13 for a description of automatic thoughts in image form).

Automatic thoughts can be evaluated according to their *validity* and their *utility*. The most common type of automatic thought is distorted in some way and occurs despite objective evidence to the contrary. A second type of automatic thought is accurate, but the *conclusion* the patient draws may be distorted. For example, "I didn't do what I promised [my roommate]" is a valid thought, but the conclusion "Therefore, I'm a bad person," is not.

A third type of automatic thought is also accurate but decidedly dysfunctional. For example, Sally was studying for an exam and thought, "It's going to take me hours to finish this. I'll be up until 3:00 A.M." This thought was undoubtedly accurate, but it increased her anxiety and decreased her concentration and motivation. A reasonable response to this thought would address its *utility*. "It's true it will take a long time to finish this, but I can do it; I've done it before. Dwelling on how long it will take makes me feel miserable, and I won't concentrate as well. It'll probably take even longer to finish. It would be better to concentrate on finishing one part at a time and giving myself credit for having finished it." Evaluating the validity and/or utility of automatic thoughts and adaptively responding to them generally produces a positive shift in affect.

To summarize, automatic thoughts coexist with a more manifest stream of thoughts, arise spontaneously, and are not based on reflection or deliberation. People are usually more aware of the associated emotion but, with a little training, they can become aware of their thinking. The thoughts relevant to personal problems are associated with *specific* emotions, depending on their content and meaning. They are often brief and fleeting, in shorthand form, and may occur in verbal and/or imaginal form. People usually accept their automatic thoughts as true, without reflection or evaluation. Identifying, evaluating, and responding to automatic thoughts (in a more adaptive way) usually produces a positive shift in affect.

EXPLAINING AUTOMATIC THOUGHTS TO PATIENTS

It is desirable to explain automatic thoughts by using the patient's own examples. Chapter 3 provided a sample transcript; following is another.

THERAPIST: Now I'd like to spend a few minutes talking about the connection between thoughts and feelings. Can you think of some times this week when you felt upset?

PATIENT: Yeah. Walking to class this morning.

T: What emotion were you feeling: sad? anxious? angry?

P: Sad.

T: What was going through your mind?

P: I was looking at these other students, talking or playing frisbee, hanging out on the lawn.

T: What was going through your mind when you saw them?

P: I'll never be like them.

T: Okay. You just identified what we call an *automatic thought*. Everyone has them. They're thoughts that just seem to pop in our heads. We're not deliberately trying to think about them; that's why we call them automatic. Most of the time, they're real quick and we're much more aware of the emotion—in this case, sadness—than we are of the thoughts. Lots of times the thoughts are distorted in some way. But we react *as if* they're true.

P: Hmmm.

T: What we'll do is to teach you to identify your automatic thoughts and then to evaluate them to see just how accurate they are. For example, in a minute we'll evaluate the thought, "I'll never be like those students." What do you think would happen to your emotions if you discovered that your thought wasn't true—that when your depression lifts you'll realize that you *are* like the other students?

P: I'd feel better.

Here the therapist suggests an alternative scenario in order to illustrate the cognitive model. Later in the session, he uses Socratic questioning to examine the thought with the patient so she can develop her own adaptive response. In the next portion, he has Sally write down the automatic thought, emphasizing the cognitive model. (See Figure 6.1.)

T: Let's get that down on paper. When you have the thought, "I'll never be like those students," you feel sad. Do you see how what you're thinking influences how you feel?

P: Uh huh.

T: That's what we call the *cognitive model*. What we'll do in therapy is to

| Thoughts | → | Feelings |

What you think influences how you feel.
Sometimes your thinking is not right or is just partially right.

| Thought | | Feeling |

| I'll never be like those students. | → | Sad |

Steps in Therapy
1. Identify automatic thoughts.
2. Evaluate and respond to automatic thoughts.
3. Do problem-solving if thoughts are true.

FIGURE 6.1. Sally's notes from Session 1.

teach you to identify your automatic thoughts when you notice your mood changing. That's the first step. We'll keep practicing it, until it's easy. Then you'll learn how to evaluate your thoughts and change your thinking if it's not completely correct. Is that clear?

P: I think so.

T: How about if we get that down on paper? Step 1: Identify automatic thoughts; Step 2: Evaluate and respond to thoughts. Could you tell me back in your own words about the relationship between thoughts and feelings?

P: Sometimes I have thoughts that are wrong and these thoughts make me feel bad. . . . But what if the thoughts are right?

T: Good point. Then we'll do some problem-solving or find out what's so bad about it if they *are* right. My guess, though, is that we'll find a lot of errors in your thinking because you *are* depressed and negative; negative thinking is always part of depression. In any case, we'll figure out together whether your interpretations are wrong. Now, can you think of any other time this week when you felt upset so we can try to identify more automatic thoughts?

At the end of this session, the therapist checks again to ascertain how well the patient seems to understand the cognitive model.

T: To review a bit, could you tell me what you now understand about the relationship between thoughts and feelings?

P: Well, sometimes automatic thoughts just pop in my head and I accept them as true. And then I feel . . . whatever: sad, worried—

T: Good. How about for homework this week if you look for some of these automatic thoughts?

P: Okay.

T: Why do you think I'm suggesting this?

P: Because sometimes my thoughts aren't true and if I can figure out what I'm thinking, I can change it around and feel better.

T: That's right. Now how about if you write this assignment down: Whenever I notice a change in mood or my mood is getting worse, ask myself . . . (*The patient writes it down.*) Now what was that $64,000 question?

P: What was just going through my mind?

T: Good! Get that down.

ELICITING AUTOMATIC THOUGHTS

The skill of learning to identify automatic thoughts is analogous to learning any other skill. Some patients (and therapists) catch on quite easily and quickly. Others need much more guidance and practice to identify automatic thoughts and images. The next two sections describe procedures for eliciting automatic thoughts (summarized in Figure 6.2).

The first method is to identify automatic thoughts the patient is having in the session itself. The second method is to elicit the automatic thoughts a patient has had about a problematic situation between sessions through recall, imagery, role-playing, or hypothesizing.

Eliciting Automatic Thoughts That Arise in Session

An opportune time to elicit a patient's automatic thought is when the therapist notices an affect shift in session.

T: Sally, I just noticed a change in your eyes. What just went through your mind?

It is vital to be alert to both verbal and nonverbal cues from the patient, so as to be able to elicit "hot cognitions"—that is, important automatic thoughts and images that arise in the therapy session itself and are associated with a change or increase in emotion. These hot cognitions may be about the patient herself ("I'm such a failure"), the therapist ("He doesn't understand me"), or the subject under discussion ("It's not fair that I have so much to do"). Eliciting the hot cognitions are important because they often are of critical importance in conceptualization. Generally, these affect-laden thoughts are the most important to work with. In addition, these hot cognitions may undermine the patient's

TECHNIQUES TO MODIFY AUTOMATIC THOUGHTS

Basic question:

What was going through your mind just then?

To identify automatic thoughts:

1. Ask this question when you notice a shift in (or intensification of) affect during a session.
2. Have the patient describe a problematic situation or a time during which she experienced an affect shift and ask the above question.
3. If needed, have the patient use imagery to describe the specific situation or time in detail (as if it is happening now) and then ask the above question.
4. If needed or desired, have the patient role-play a specific interaction with you and then ask the above question.

Other questions to elicit automatic thoughts:

1. What do you guess you were thinking about?
2. Do you think you could have been thinking about _____ or _____?
   (Therapist provides a couple of plausible possibilities.)
3. Were you imagining something that might happen or remembering something that did?
4. What did this situation mean to you? (Or say about you?)
5. Were you thinking _____? (Therapist provides a thought opposite to the expected response.)

FIGURE 6.2. Summary of techniques to identify automatic thoughts. Copyright 1993 by Judith S. Beck, Ph.D.

motivation or sense of adequacy or worth. They may interfere with the patient's concentration in session. Finally, they may interfere with the therapeutic relationship. Identifying automatic thoughts on the spot gives the patient the opportunity to test and respond to the thoughts immediately so as to facilitate the work in the rest of the session.

How does the therapist know when a patient has experienced an affect shift? He is on the alert for nonverbal cues such as changes in facial expression, tightening of muscles, shifts in posture, or hand gestures. Verbal cues include change in tone, pitch, volume, or pace. Having noticed a change, the therapist infers an affect shift and checks it out by asking the patient what just went through her mind. If the patient is unable to report a thought, the therapist may choose to jog her memory by having her focus on her emotion and physiological reaction.

T: Sally, what's going through your mind right now?

P: I'm not sure.

T: How are you feeling right now?

P: I don't know. Sad, I guess.

T: Where do you feel the sadness?

P: In my chest. And behind my eyes.

T: So, when I asked, "How's school going?" you felt sad. Any idea what you were thinking about?

P: I think it was about my economics class. I was thinking about getting back my exam.

T: What were you thinking? Or did you imagine something?

P: Yeah. I pictured a "C" at the top, in red ink.

With a little gentle persistence, Sally was able to report her image. Had focusing on the emotion *not* helped, the therapist might have chosen to change the subject so as not to make Sally feel that she was being interrogated or to reduce the possibility of Sally's viewing herself as a failure for not being able to identify her automatic thought.

T: No big deal. How about if we continue on with the agenda.

On the other hand, it might be wise to pursue this hot cognition. Although it is more desirable to get the patient to identify her specific thoughts rather than speculating about them, a number of questions can be useful when she is unable to do so. The therapist might ask Sally to make a guess or he might pose plausible possibilities. He could specifically ask about an image or ask for the meaning of the situation to her. Or he could suggest a specific thought which is actually the *opposite* of what he conjectures her thought was.

T: What went through your mind when I asked, "How's school going?" and you felt sad?

P: I don't know. I really don't. I just felt so down.

T: If you had to take a guess, what would you guess you were thinking about? [Or, do you think you could have been thinking about school, or about your work, or about therapy? Or, could you have been picturing something in your mind? Or, what did it mean to you that I asked you about school? Or, were you thinking how great everything is going?]

Identifying Automatic Thoughts in a Specific Situation

These same questions can be used to help the patient identify automatic thoughts she had between sessions. Again, the therapist first tries the standard question ("What was going through your mind?") when the patient describes a problematic situation. Often the patient is helped by the therapist's request for a more detailed description of what had been going on.

T: So, you were sitting in class, and you suddenly felt nervous? What was going through your mind?

P: I don't know.

T: What was happening?

P: The professor was explaining what the requirements of the paper were, and the guy next to me whispered a question to me about when it was due.

T: So, this guy whispered while the professor was explaining? And you felt nervous?

P: Yes, I know, I was thinking, "What did she say? What did I miss? Now I won't know what to do."

If verbally describing the situation is insufficient to elicit the automatic thoughts, the therapist asks the patient to imagine the specific situation as if it is happening *right now*. He encourages her to use as much detail as possible, speaking in the present tense.

T: Sally, can you imagine that you're back in the class *right now*, the professor is talking, the student next to you is whispering, you're feeling nervous. . . . Describe it to me in as much detail as you can, as if it's happening right now. How big is the class? Where are you sitting? Where is the professor? What is she saying? What are you doing, and so on.

P: I'm in my economics class. The professor is standing in front of the class. Let's see, I was sitting about three-quarters of the way back, I was listening pretty hard—

T: So, "I'm sitting three-quarters of the way back, I'm listening pretty hard. . . ." (*Guiding the patient to speak as if it's happening right at the moment.*)

P: She's saying something about what topics we can choose, a macro-economic view of the economy or . . . something, and then this guy on my left leans over and whispers, "When's the paper due?"

T: And what's going through your mind right now?

P: What did she say? What did I miss? Now I won't know what to do.

The therapist helps the patient reexperience the situation as if it is happening right then. When he notices that the patient seems to be reverting to past tense, he gently guides her back to the present tense so the experience is more immediate. Likewise, if a patient has difficulty identifying automatic thoughts in an interpersonal situation, the therapist can help recreate the situation through role-play. The patient describes who said what verbally, then the patient plays herself while the therapist plays the other person in the interaction.

T: So, you were feeling down as you were talking to your classmate about the assignment?

P: Yes.

T: What was going through your mind as you were talking to her?

P: (*Pauses.*) . . . I don't know. I was just really down.

T: Can you tell me what you said to her and what she said to you?

P: (*Describes verbal exchange.*)

T: How about if we try a role-play? I'll be the classmate and you be you.

P: Okay.

T: While we're recreating the situation, see if you can figure out what's going through your mind.

P: (*Nods.*)

T: Okay, you start. What do you say first?

P: Karen, can I ask you a question?

T: Sure, but can you call me later? I've got to run to my next class.

P: It's fast. I just missed part of what Dr. Smith said about our paper.

T: I'm really in a hurry now. Call me after 7:00, okay? Bye. . . . Okay, out of role-play. Were you aware of what was going through your mind?

P: Yeah. I was thinking that she was too busy for me, that she didn't really want to help me, and I wouldn't know what to do.

T: You had the thoughts, "She's too busy for me." "She doesn't really want to help me." "I won't know what to do."

P: Yes.

T: And those thoughts made you feel sad?

P: Yeah.

If the patient is still unable to report her thoughts, the therapist might move onto something else or use the more specific questions outlined in Figure 6.2.

Identifying Additional Automatic Thoughts

It is important to continue questioning the patient even after she reports an initial automatic thought. This additional questioning may bring to light other important thoughts.

T: So when you got the test back, you thought, "I should have done better. I should have studied harder." What else went through your mind?

P: Everyone else probably did better than me.

T: Then what?

P: I was thinking, "I shouldn't even be here. I'm such a failure."

The therapist should be aware that the patient may, in addition, have other automatic thoughts not about the same situation itself but about her *reaction* to that situation. She may perceive her emotion, behavior, or physiological reaction in a negative way.

T: So you had the thought, "I might embarrass myself," and you felt anxious? Then what happened?

P: My heart started beating real fast and I thought, "What's wrong with me?"

T: And you felt . . . ?

P: More anxious.

T: And then?

P: I thought, "I'll never feel okay."

T: And you felt . . . ?

P: Sad and hopeless.

Note that the patient first had automatic thoughts about a specific situation (volunteering in class). Then she had thoughts about her anxiety and her bodily reaction. In many cases, these secondary emotional reactions can be quite distressing and significantly compound an already upsetting situation. In order to work most efficiently, it is important to determine at which point the patient was *most* distressed (before, during, or after a given incident) and what her automatic thoughts were at that point. The patient may have had distressing automatic thoughts in *anticipation* of a situation ("What if she yells at me?"), *during* the situation ("She thinks I'm stupid"), and/or at a *later* point, reflecting on what had happened ("I can't do anything right; I should never have tried").

IDENTIFYING THE PROBLEMATIC SITUATION

Sometimes, in addition to being unable to identify automatic thoughts associated with a given emotion, a patient has difficulty even identifying the one situation or issue that is most troublesome to her (or which part is the most upsetting). When this happens, the therapist can help her pinpoint the most problematic situation by proposing a number of upsetting problems, asking the patient hypothetically to eliminate one problem, and determining how much relief the patient feels. Once a specific situation has been identified, the automatic thoughts are more easily uncovered.

T: (*Summarizing.*) So, you've been very upset for the past few days and you're not sure why and you're having trouble identifying your thoughts—you just feel upset most of the time. Is that right?

P: Yes. I just don't know why I'm so upset all the time.

T: What kinds of things have you been thinking about?

P: Well, school for one. And I'm not getting along well with my roommate. And then I tried to get hold of my mother again and I couldn't reach her, and, I don't know, just everything.

T: So, there is a problem with school, with your roommate, with reaching your mom . . . anything else?

P: Yeah. I haven't been feeling too well. I'm afraid I might be getting sick just before this big paper is due.

T: Which of these situations bothers you the most—school, roommate, reaching your mom, feeling sick?

P: Oh, I don't know. I'm worried about all of them.

T: Let's jot these four things down. Now let's say hypothetically we could completely eliminate the feeling sick problem, let's say you now feel physically fine, how anxious are you now?

P: About the same.

T: Okay. Say, hypothetically, you do reach your mom right away after therapy and everything's fine with her. How do you feel now?

P: A little bit better. Not that much.

T: Okay. Let's say the school problem—what is the school problem?

P: I have a paper due next week.

T: Okay, let's say you've just handed the paper in early, and you're feeling good about it. Now how do you feel?

P: That would be a great relief, if that paper were done and I thought I'd done well.

T: So it sounds as if it's the paper that is the most distressing situation.

P: Yeah. I think so.

T: Now just to make sure. . . . If you still had the paper to do, but the roommate problem disappeared, how would you feel?

P: Not that good. I think it *is* the paper that's bothering me the most.

T: In a moment, we'll focus on the school problem, but first I'd like to review how we figured it out so you'll be able to do it yourself in the future.

P: Well, you had me list all the things I was worried about and pretend to solve them one by one.

T: And then you were able to see which one would give you the most relief if it had been resolved.

P: Yeah.

[Therapist and patient then focus on the school problem; they identify and respond to automatic thoughts and do some problem-solving.]

The same process can be used in helping the patient to determine which *part* of a seemingly overwhelming problem is most distressing.

T: So you've been pretty upset about your roommate. What *specifically* has been bothering you?

P: Oh, I don't know. Everything.

T: Can you name some things?

P: Well, she's been taking my food and not replacing it. Not in a malicious way, but it still bothers me. And she's got a boyfriend and whenever she talks about him, it reminds me that I don't have one. And she's messy; she leaves stuff all around. . . . And she's kind of inconsiderate. She forgets to give me phone messages and things like that.

T: Anything else?

P: Those are the major ones.

T: Okay, we've done this before. Let me read these back to you so you can figure out which one bothers you the most. If you can't, we'll hypothetically eliminate them one by one and see which one makes the biggest difference in how you feel. Okay?

DIFFERENTIATING BETWEEN AUTOMATIC THOUGHTS AND INTERPRETATIONS

When the therapist asks for the patient's automatic thoughts, he is seeking the *actual* words or images that have gone through her mind. Until they have learned to recognize these thoughts, many patients report *interpretations*, which may or may not reflect the actual thoughts. In the following transcript, the therapist guides the patient to report her thoughts.

T: When you saw that woman in the cafeteria, what went through your mind?

P: I think I was denying my real feelings.

T: What were you actually thinking?

P: I'm not sure what you mean.

In this exchange, the patient reported an *interpretation* of what she was feeling and thinking. Below, the therapist tries again, by focusing on and heightening her emotion.

T: When you saw her, what emotion did you feel?

P: I think I was just denying my feelings.

T: Uh huh. What feelings were you denying?

P: I'm not sure.

T: When you saw her, did you feel happy? Excited? (*Supplying an emotion opposite to the expected one to jog her recall.*)

P: No, not at all.

T: Can you remember walking in the cafeteria and seeing her? Can you picture that in your mind?

P: Uh huh.

T: What are you feeling?

P: Sad, I think.

T: As you look at her, what goes through your mind?

P: I feel really sad, an emptiness in the pit of my stomach. (*Reporting an emotion and a physiological reaction instead of an automatic thought.*)

T: What's going through your mind now?

P: She's really smart. I'm nothing compared to her.

T: (*Jotting down the thoughts.*) Okay. Anything else?

P: No. I just walked over to the table and started talking to my friend.

DIFFERENTIATING BETWEEN USEFUL AND RELATIVELY LESS USEFUL AUTOMATIC THOUGHTS

Until the patient learns to recognize the *specific* automatic thoughts that distress her, she may report a number of thoughts. Some thoughts are simply descriptive and innocuous or irrelevant to a problem. *Relevant* automatic thoughts are usually associated with marked distress. As in the previous section, the therapist tries to determine which thought or thoughts will be most productive to focus on.

T: So you were feeling pretty sad when you hung up the phone. What was going through your mind right then?

P: Well, my friend from high school is really doing well. She's got a job, she's hanging out with a lot of our friends. She gets to use her family's car so she's not hemmed in. Sometimes I wish I were more like her. She's doing really good. I'm such a loser—.

T: Did you have that thought "I'm such a loser," as you hung up the phone?

P: (*Nods.*)

T: Anything else go through your mind just then?

P: No, just that I'm a loser. I'll never be like her.

SPECIFYING AUTOMATIC THOUGHTS EMBEDDED IN DISCOURSE

Patients need to learn to specify the actual words that go through their minds in order to evaluate them effectively. Following are some examples of embedded thoughts versus actual words:

Embedded expressions	*Actual automatic thoughts*
I guess I was wondering if he likes me.	Does he like me?

(*cont.*)

| I don't know if going to
the professor would be
a waste of time. | It'll probably be a waste
time if I go. |
| I couldn't get myself to start
reading. | I can't do this. |

The therapist gently leads the patient to identify the *actual* words that went through her mind.

T: So when you turned bright red in class, what went through your mind?

P: I guess I was wondering if he thought I was strange.

T: Can you recall the exact words you were thinking?

P: (*Puzzled.*) I'm not sure what you mean.

T: Were you thinking, "I guess I was wondering if he thought I was strange," or were you thinking, "Does he think I'm strange?"

P: Oh I see, the second one. Or actually I think it was, "He probably thinks I'm strange."

CHANGING THE FORM OF TELEGRAPHIC
OR QUESTION THOUGHTS

Patients often report thoughts that are not fully spelled out. As it is difficult to evaluate such a telegraphic thought, the therapist guides the patient to express the thought more fully.

T: What went through your mind when the paper was announced?

P: Uh, oh. I just thought, "Uh, oh."

T: Can you spell the thought out? "Uh, oh" means . . .

P: I'll never get the work done in time. I have too much to do.

If the patient had been unable to spell out her thought, the therapist might have tried supplying an opposite thought: "Did 'Uh, oh' mean 'That's really good'?"

Automatic thoughts are sometimes expressed in the form of a question, making evaluation difficult. Therefore, the therapist guides the patient in expressing the thought in a statement form prior to helping her evaluate it.

T: So you felt anxious? What was going through your mind right then?

P: I was thinking, "Will I pass the test?"

T: Okay, now before we evaluate that thought, let's see if we can restate it in the form of a statement, so we can work with it more easily. Were you thinking you probably would or wouldn't pass the test?

P: That I wouldn't.

T: Okay. So can we rephrase your thought as, "I might not pass the test"?

   Another example follows:

T: So you had the thought, "What will happen to me [if I get more and more nervous]?" What are you *afraid* could happen?

P: I don't know . . lose control, I guess.

T: Okay, let's look at that thought, "I could lose control."

   In the previous example, the therapist leads the patient into revealing precisely what she fears. In the next example, the patient initially has difficulty identifying the fear behind her automatic thought, so the therapist tries several different questions to identify the thought:

T: So you thought, "What next?" What did you think would happen next?

P: I don't know.

T: Were you afraid something specific might happen?

P: I'm not sure.

T: What's the worst thing that *could* happen in this situation?

P: Ummm . . . that I'd get kicked out of school.

T: Do you think that was what you were afraid would happen at the time?

   The box illustrates other examples of how questions can be restated in order to be evaluated more effectively.

Question	*Statement*
Will I be able to cope?	I won't be able to cope.
Can I stand it if she leaves?	I won't be able to stand it if she leaves.
What if I can't do it?	I'll lose my job if I can't do it.
What if she gets mad at me?	She'll hurt me if she gets mad at me.

(*cont.*)

How will I get through it?	I won't be able to get through it.
What if I can't change?	I'll be miserable forever if I can't change.
Why did this happen to me?	This shouldn't have happened to me.

TEACHING PATIENTS TO IDENTIFY
AUTOMATIC THOUGHTS

As described in Chapter 4, the therapist can begin teaching the patient the skill of identifying automatic thoughts even at the first session. Here the therapist has just demonstrated the cognitive model, using the patient's own examples.

T: Sally, when you notice your mood changing or getting worse in the next week, could you stop and ask yourself, "What is going through my mind right now?"

P: Yeah.

T: Maybe you could jot down a few of these thoughts on a piece of paper?

P: Sure.

In later sessions, the therapist might also explicitly teach the patient other techniques if the basic question ("What's going through your mind right now?") is not helping enough.

T: Sometimes you may not be able to tell what you were thinking. So either at the time or later you can try what we just did here in session. Replay the scene as vividly as you can in your imagination, as if it's happening again, and concentrate on how you're feeling. Then ask yourself, "What's going through my mind?" Do you think you could do that? Or should we practice it again?

P: I'll give it a try.

Again, if asking the basic questions and trying the imagery technique are not sufficient, the therapist might explicitly teach the patient to hypothesize about her thoughts. This method is a second choice because it is more likely the patient will report a later interpretation instead of her actual thoughts at the time.

T: If you still have trouble figuring out what was going through your mind, here are some other questions [see Figure 6.2] you can ask yourself.

P: Okay.

T: First question: If I had to, what would I guess I was thinking about? Or, could I have been thinking about _____ or _____? Or, was I imagining something or remembering something? Or, finally, what does this situation mean to me? Or you might try to figure out what the opposite thought might be to jog your memory.

P: Okay.

T: How about trying out these questions this week if you have trouble identifying your automatic thoughts and if imagining the situation again doesn't help?

P: Fine.

To summarize, people with psychological disorders make predictable errors in their thinking. The cognitive therapist teaches patients to identify their dysfunctional thinking, then to evaluate and modify it. The process starts with the recognition of specific automatic thoughts in specific situations. Identifying automatic thoughts is a skill that comes easily and naturally to some patients and is more difficult for others. The therapist needs to listen closely to ensure that a patient is reporting actual thoughts and may need to vary his questioning if the patient does not readily identify her thoughts. The next chapter clarifies, among other things, the difference between automatic thoughts and emotions.

Chapter 7

IDENTIFYING EMOTIONS

Emotions are of primary importance to the cognitive therapist. After all, a major goal of therapy is symptom relief, a reduction in a patient's level of distress when she modifies her dysfunctional thinking.

Intense negative emotion is painful and may be dysfunctional if it interferes with a patient's capacity to think clearly, solve problems, act effectively, or gain satisfaction. Patients with a psychiatric disorder often experience an intensity of emotion that is excessive or inappropriate to the situation. Sally, for example, felt enormous guilt and then sadness when she had to cancel a minor social event with her roommate. She was also extremely anxious about going to a professor for help.

Although the therapist may recognize the excessiveness or inappropriateness of an emotion, he refrains from labeling it as such, especially early in therapy. Rather, he *acknowledges* and *empathizes* with how the patient feels. He does not challenge or dispute the patient's emotions but rather focuses on evaluating the dysfunctional thoughts and beliefs underlying her distress in order to reduce her dysphoria.

The therapist does not analyze *all* situations in which the patient feels dysphoric, however; cognitive therapy aims to reduce the emotional distress that is related to *misinterpretations* of a situation. "Normal" negative emotions are as much a part of the richness of life as positive emotions and serve as important a function as does physical pain, alerting us to a potential problem that may need to be addressed.

In addition, the therapist seeks to increase the patient's *positive* emotions through discussion (usually relatively brief) of the patient's interests, positive events that occurred during the week, positive memories, and so forth. He often suggests homework assignments aimed at increasing the number of activities in which the patient is likely to experience mastery and pleasure (see Chapter 12).

This chapter explains how to differentiate automatic thoughts from

94

emotions, how to distinguish among emotions, how to label emotions, and how to rate the intensity of emotions.

DISTINGUISHING AUTOMATIC THOUGHTS FROM EMOTIONS

Many patients do not clearly understand the difference between what they are thinking and what they are feeling emotionally. The therapist tries to make sense of the patient's experience and shares his understanding with the patient. He continually and subtly helps the patient view her experiences through the cognitive model.

The therapist organizes the material the patient presents into the categories of the cognitive model: situation, automatic thought, and reaction (emotion, behavior, and physiological response). It is important to be alert to occasions when the patient confuses thoughts and emotions. At these times, based on the flow of the session, their goals, and the collaboration, the therapist decides whether to ignore the confusion altogether or to address it later or right at the time (either subtly or explicitly).

At times, mislabeling a thought as a feeling is relatively unimportant in a given context, and it is better to address the confusion when discussing something else later on, if ever. In this case, the therapist ignores the confusion altogether.

THERAPIST: You mentioned when we set the agenda that you wanted to talk about the phone call you had with your brother.

PATIENT: Yeah. I called him a couple of nights ago, and I felt like he really didn't want to talk. He sounded kind of distant. I was feeling like he didn't really care if I had called or not.

T: If it were true that he didn't really care if you had called or not, what would that mean to you?

In this case, the therapist wants to uncover the underlying belief and so ignores the patient's verbal mix-up of feeling and thought. They proceed to evaluate and modify a key dysfunctional assumption.

In another session, the therapist views the confusion as important. He judges, however, that helping to clarify the confusion at the time might interrupt the flow of the session or interfere with his goal for the session (or that segment of the session). In this case, he finishes the topic at hand and returns to make the distinction between thoughts and emotion later.

T: I want to get back to something we talked about a few minutes ago. Do you remember when you were telling me that you knew you should go to the library last night but you didn't feel like going?

P: Yeah.

T: Actually, my guess is that you had a *thought* like, "I don't want to go," or "I don't feel like going." Is that right?

P: Yeah, I thought, "I don't feel like going."

T: What *emotion* went along with the thought, "I don't feel like going"?

P: I was a little anxious, I guess.

In many cases, the therapist subtly corrects the patient who has confused thoughts with emotions.

P: I was lying in bed, staring at the ceiling, feeling like I'd never be able to get up and that I'd be late for class.

T: So you were lying in bed and you had a couple of thoughts: I'll never be able to get up. I'll be late for class.

P: Yes.

T: And how did those thoughts make you feel emotionally?

Finally, the therapist occasionally decides to make a sharp distinction for the patient, judging that it is important to do so at the time and that the flow of the session will not be unduly interrupted or important data forgotten.

T: Were there any times this week when you thought about doing therapy homework?

P: Yeah, a few times.

T: Can you remember one time specifically?

P: Last night, after dinner, I was cleaning up, and I realized our appointment was today.

T: What was going through your mind right then?

P: Oh, I was feeling like it's no use. It probably won't help.

T: Those are good thoughts. We'll get back to evaluating them in a minute, but first I'd like to review the difference between thoughts and feelings. Okay?

P: Sure.

T: Feelings are what you feel *emotionally*—like sadness, anger, anxiety, and so on. Thoughts are *ideas* that you have; you think them either in words or in pictures or images. Is that clear to you?

P: I think so.

T: So let's get back to the time last night when you thought about doing therapy homework. What emotion were you feeling?

P: Sad, I think.

T: And what thoughts did you have?

P: "This is no use. I'll never get better."

T: So you had the thoughts, "This is no use. I'll never get better," and those thoughts made you feel sad. Is that right?

P: Yeah.

In the examples in the transcript, the patient initially labeled thoughts as feelings. At times, the patient does the reverse, that is, labels an emotion as a thought:

T: As you walked into your empty dorm room, Sally, what went through your mind?

P: Sad, lonely, real down.

T: So you felt very sad and lonely and down. What thought or image made you feel that way?

IMPORTANCE OF DISTINGUISHING AMONG EMOTIONS

The therapist is continuously conceptualizing or reformulating the patient's problems, trying to understand the patient's experience and point of view. He tries to figure out how the patient's underlying beliefs gave rise to specific automatic thoughts in a specific situation and influenced the patient's emotions and behavior. The connection among the thoughts, emotion, and behavior should make sense to the therapist. He investigates further when the patient reports an emotion *that does not seem to match* the content of her automatic thought, as in the transcript below.

T: How did you feel when your mother didn't call you back right away?

P: I was sad.

T: What was going through your mind?

P: What if something happened to her? Maybe there's something wrong.

T: And you felt sad?

P: Yes.

T: I'm a little confused because those sound more like anxious thoughts. Was there anything else going on through your mind?

P: I'm not sure.

T: How about if we have you imagine the scene. You said you were sitting by the phone, waiting for her call?

[The therapist helps the patient vividly recall the scene in imagery form.]

P: And then I thought, "What if something happened? Maybe there's something wrong."

T: What happens next?

P: I'm looking at the phone, and I get teary.

T: What's going through your mind right now?

P: If anything happened to Mom, there would be no one left who cares.

T: There would be no one left who cares. How does that thought make you feel?

P: Sad. Real sad.

This interchange started with a discrepancy. The therapist was alert and picked up a possible inconsistency between the content of the automatic thought and the emotion associated with it. He was then able to help the patient retrieve a key automatic thought by using imaginal recall. Had he chosen to focus on the anxious thoughts, he may have missed the patient's more central concern. Although it may have been helpful to focus on a less central thought, finding and working with *key* automatic thoughts usually speed up therapy.

DIFFICULTY IN LABELING EMOTIONS

Most patients easily and correctly label their emotions. Some, however, display a relatively impoverished vocabulary for emotions; others understand emotional labels intellectually but have difficulty labeling their own specific emotions. In either of these two cases, it is useful to have the patient link her emotional reactions in specific situations to their labels. Devising an "Emotion Chart" such as the one in Figure 7.1 helps the patient learn to label her emotions more effectively.

T: I'd like to spend a few minutes talking about different emotions so we can both understand better how you feel in different situations. Okay?

Angry	Sad	Anxious
1. Brother says he's leaving to see friends.	1. Mom does not return phone call.	1. Raising hand in class.
2. Roommate does not return book.	2. Dorm meeting—no one pays attention to me.	2. Writing economics paper.
3. Roommate plays music too loud.	3. "C" on midterm.	3. Asking friend to go to dinner.

FIGURE 7.1. Sally's emotion chart.

P: Sure.

T: Can you remember a time when you felt angry?

P: Uh, yeah. . . . When my brother came home from college and acted all high and mighty. . . . He didn't want to spend any time with me.

T: Do you remember a specific scene?

P: Yes. It was Christmas vacation. I hadn't seen him since Thanksgiving. I thought we would hang out together that first day he got home, but he announced that he was leaving right away to go see his friends.

T: And what was going through your mind?

P: Who does he think he is? He thinks he's so great just because he's in college now.

T: And you felt—

P: Mad.

The therapist has the patient recall a *specific* event in which the patient felt a given emotion. From her description, it sounds as if the patient has correctly identified her emotion. The therapist, however, wants to make sure so he asks her to identify her automatic thoughts. The content of the automatic thoughts does match the stated emotion.

Next, the therapist asks the patient to recall two more occasions when she felt angry. This interchange occurs fairly quickly and the therapist does not ask for specific thoughts because he is reasonably certain from her description that she is accurately labeling the emotion. He follows up with an assignment.

T: Let's have you jot down these three situations in which you felt angry. Here, let's make columns and label the first one "angry." Can you jot down a couple of words that will describe the three situations? [See Figure 7.1.]

P: (*Does so.*)

T: We're a little short on time. Suppose we label these other two columns "sad" and "anxious." Would you see if you can think of specific situations when you felt these emotions and jot them down at home? Do you think you could do it without too much trouble?

P: Yeah, I think so.

T: (*Checking whether the patient remembers rationale for the assignment.*) Do you remember why it's worth spending this time to differentiate your emotions?

P: Well, sometimes I'm not sure how I feel or what is bothering me, so doing this should help.

T: Right. And maybe you could refer to this sheet during the week when you notice you feel upset and try to figure out which emotion you *are* feeling. Okay?

P: Okay.

T: Let's have you write these things down on your homework sheet, to finish this "Emotion Chart" and refer to it when you're upset.

Again, with most patients, it is not necessary to use this technique to differentiate emotions. Others may benefit from a quick discussion along the above lines. A few might profit from a list of negative emotions (see Figure 7.2) and a brief discussion.

Sad, down, lonely, unhappy

Anxious, worried, fearful, scared, tense

Angry, mad, irritated, annoyed

Ashamed, embarrassed, humiliated

Disappointed

Jealous, envious

Guilty

Hurt

Suspicious

FIGURE 7.2. Negative emotions.

DIFFICULTY IN RATING DEGREE OF EMOTION

It is important for patients not only to identify their emotions but also to quantify the *degree* of emotion they are experiencing. Some have dysfunctional beliefs about emotion itself, for example, believing that if they feel a small amount of distress, it will increase and become intolerable. Learning to rate the intensity of emotions will aid the patient in testing this belief.

In addition, it is important to assess whether questioning and adaptively responding to a thought or belief have been effective. The therapist and patient judge whether a cognition requires further intervention by roughly measuring the drop in intensity of the emotion. Therapists who neglect to assess the change in distress may mistakenly assume that an intervention has been successful and proceed to the next thought or problem prematurely. Or the opposite may happen; they may continue discussing an automatic thought or belief, not realizing that the patient is no longer distressed by it.

Finally, gauging the intensity of an emotion in a given situation helps the patient and therapist determine whether that situation warrants closer scrutiny. A situation that is relatively less emotionally laden may be less valuable to discuss than one that is more distressing to the patient, where important beliefs may have been activated.

Most patients learn to judge the intensity of an emotion fairly easily, without a visual aid.

T: How did you feel when your friend said, "Sorry, I don't have time now"?

P: Pretty sad, I guess.

T: If 100% is the saddest you ever felt or could imagine feeling, and 0 is completely *not* sad, how sad did you feel right when he said, "Sorry, I don't have time now"?

P: About 75%.

Some patients have difficulty putting a specific number to the intensity. The therapist may then draw a scale:

0%	25%	50%	75%	100%
Not sad at all	Somewhat sad	Medium sad	Quite sad	Saddest I have been or could imagine being

T: Sometimes it's easier to remember if you imagine yourself back in the situation. (*Asks the patient to "relive" the experience as if it is happening now.*) Now take a look at this scale. How sad do you think you felt after the meeting? Somewhat sad? Medium sad? Quite sad?

P: Oh, somewhere between quite sad and the saddest I've ever been.

T: Somewhere between 75% and 100% sad? Which number is it closer to?

P: Oh, I guess 80% sad.

If the patient *still* has difficulty rating the intensity of her emotions, the therapist may consider helping the patient to build an idiosyncratic Emotional Intensity Scale to use as a guide for future ratings (Figure 7.3). The therapist chooses the patient's predominant emotion and provides or elicits a rationale.

T: Sometimes making a list of specific situations that were associated with an emotion can help. But, first, do you know why I'm even emphasizing this? Why might it be important to rate how intense your emotion is?

P: You said last week that it's one way to know if it's worth discussing something. And also to know if answering back a thought has helped.

Degree of emotion/anxiety	Situations
0%	Watching movie on TV last Saturday
10%	Wondering if I'd be late to therapy today
20%	Pain in side: appendicitis?
30%	Wondering why mom called unexpectedly
40%	Thinking about how much work I have to do
50%	Volunteering in class when I'm sure of the answer
60%	Thinking about going to the teaching assistant
70%	Talking to friends about life after graduation
80%	Volunteering in class when I'm unsure of my answer
90%	The night before my economics midterm
100%	My father's car accident

FIGURE 7.3. Sally's emotional intensity scale.

T: Okay. Now let's make a list of situations in which you felt anxious. What is the *most* anxious you've ever felt or could imagine feeling?

P: Uh . . . that probably was when my father was in a car accident, and I thought he was going to die.

T: (*Writes or has the patient write "Father's car accident" at bottom of paper.*) Now when was a time when you weren't the least bit anxious?

P: Oh, I guess on Saturday when I was watching a movie on television.

T: We'll put that at the bottom of the page. (*Does so.*) Okay, how about a situation in between?

P: Well, yesterday, when I thought about how much work I had to do.

T: (*Writes this item near the middle.*) Okay, another time that you were anxious.

P: When I had a sharp pain in my side, and I was worried it could be appendicitis.

T: Okay. Were you more nervous when you had the pain in your side or when you were thinking how much work you had to do?

P: Thinking about my work. I was just a little nervous about the appendicitis. It turned out to be nothing anyway.

T: (*Writes "Pain in side: appendicitis" near top of the page.*) Okay, another situation?

P: Well, the night before my economics exam.

T: Where would that go?

P: Below my dad's car accident.

Therapist and patient continue in the same vein until they have collected about 10 situations of different intensities. Sometimes they need to reassess the relative intensity of a situation. Sometimes a situation is eliminated if the patient judges that it evokes the same emotional intensity as does another situation. If there is insufficient time in session to record 10 situations, the therapist can ask the patient to continue the assignment at home. When the situations are ranked from not at all anxious to most anxious, the therapist then assigns percentages in degrees of 10. He confirms with the patient that the numbers assigned roughly correspond to each situation. If not, the numbers and/or situations are revised. Next he teaches the patient how to use the scale:

T: Okay, we've got our scale now. Let's see how useful it is. Did any other situation come up this week in which you found you were anxious?

P: Yeah, last night when I remembered that I hadn't finished my therapy homework.

T: Use your new scale as a guide. About how anxious did you feel?

P: Well, a little bit more than being worried that I'd be late for therapy.

T: What number would you put on it?

P: About 15%, I guess.

T: Good. I'd like you to use this scale as a guide whenever you're trying to figure out how anxious you are. Do you see any problems with doing that?

P: No. I think it'll be easier.

USING EMOTIONAL INTENSITY TO GUIDE THERAPY

The patient may not realize which situations she should bring up for discussion in therapy. The therapist can ask her to rate the degree of distress she feels or felt in order to decide whether discussion of a given situation is likely to benefit her. In the next transcript, the therapist quickly realizes that they will probably not accomplish much by focusing on an initial situation which Sally describes:

T: How did you feel when your roommate went out with her boyfriend instead of you?

P: Sad.

T: About how sad, 0–100%?

P: Not much. Maybe 20, 25%.

T: Sounds like you didn't feel *too* bad then. Was there another time this week when you got pretty upset with her?

In summary, the therapist aims to obtain a clear picture of a situation that is upsetting to a patient. He helps her clearly differentiate her thoughts and her emotions. He empathizes with her emotions throughout this process and helps her evaluate the dysfunctional thinking that has influenced her mood.

Chapter 8

EVALUATING AUTOMATIC THOUGHTS

P atients have many thousands of thoughts a day, some dysfunctional, some not. In the interest of efficiency, the therapist selects just one or a few key thoughts to evaluate in a given session. This chapter describes how to select the most useful automatic thoughts for evaluation, how to evaluate these thoughts, and how to teach patients a system for evaluating their own thoughts.

DECIDING WHETHER TO FOCUS ON AN AUTOMATIC THOUGHT

A therapist may uncover several or many automatic thoughts in a given session. Having uncovered one, how does he decide what to do next? He has several options. He can:

1. *Focus on the automatic thought.* ("How much do you/did you believe this thought?" "How did this thought make you *feel emotionally*?" "What did you *do* after you had this thought?")
2. *Find out more about the situation associated with the automatic thought.* ("What had Karen said to you just *before* you had that thought?" "When did this happen?" "Where were you?" "Tell me more about the situation.")
3. *Explore how typical the automatic thought is.* ("How often do you have this kind of thought?" "In what situations?" "How much does this kind of thought bother you?")

(cont.)

4. *Identify other automatic thoughts and images in this same situation.* ("Anything else go through your mind?" "Any images or pictures?")

5. *Do problem-solving about the situation associated with the automatic thought.* ("What are some things you could do about this?" "How have you handled this kind of thing before?" "What do you wish you could do?")

6. *Explore the belief underlying the automatic thought.* ("If this thought is true, what would it mean to you?")

7. *Move on to another topic.* ("Okay. I think I understand that. Can you tell me what else happened this week?")

How does the therapist choose among these options? He asks himself:

1. What am I trying to accomplish in this session? Will working on this thought help us reach the therapeutic goals I have for the session?

2. What did the patient put on the agenda? Will focusing on this thought address the problem(s) she wants to work on? If not, will we have sufficient time to get to her concerns? Will she collaborate with me in evaluating this thought?

3. Is this an important thought on which to focus? Does it seem significantly distorted or dysfunctional? How typical or central is it? Will focusing on it help the patient in more than just this one situation? Will exploring it help me to conceptualize the patient better?

Sally, for example, was describing a problem she had had in the library.

THERAPIST: What went through your mind when you couldn't find the book you needed?

PATIENT: That they are so inefficient there. The system is so poor.

T: How did that thought make you feel?

P: Frustrated.

T: How frustrated?

P: 90%.

T: Then what happened?

P: I said, "To hell with it," and went back to my room and worked on my chemistry problems instead.

T: What happened to your mood then?

P: I felt better. I ended up borrowing the book from Lisa. I have to give it back to her by Monday, though.

T: So you solved the problem. Anything else important about this before we move on?

Here the therapist judges that the automatic thought, while distressing at the time, did not warrant further discussion because (1) Sally was no longer distressed by it, (2) Sally had acted in a functional way, (3) the situation was resolved, (4) there were more pressing problems on the agenda, and (5) Sally had not previously exhibited a dysfunctional pattern in this kind of situation.

FOCUSING ON AN AUTOMATIC THOUGHT

Having decided to attend to an automatic thought, the therapist tries to confirm that the thought is worth exploring by asking the following:

1. How much do you believe this thought now (0–100%)?
2. How does this thought make you feel (emotionally)?
3. How strong (0–100%) is [this emotion]?

If the degree of belief and distress is low, the therapist most likely suggests moving on to something else. If the patient believes the automatic thought strongly and is significantly distressed by it, the therapist fleshes out the picture by asking questions according to the cognitive model:

1. When did you have this thought? In what specific situation?
2. What other distressing thoughts and images did you have in this situation?
3. [Especially for anxious patients:] What did you notice, if anything, happening in your body?
4. What did you do next?

After obtaining a fuller picture, the therapist might do one or more of the following:

1. Conceptualize aloud or to himself how the thought(s) in this particular situation fit into his broader conceptualization of the patient: "Sally, could this be another example of how you consistently predict you'll fail?"
2. Use this automatic thought to reinforce the cognitive model (usually early in therapy) implicitly or explicitly; for

(cont.)

example, "So when you were in the library, trying to study, you had the thought, 'I'll never learn all of this.' This thought made you feel sad and led to your closing the book and giving up. Is that right?"

3. Help the patient evaluate and respond to the thought through Socratic questioning, as in the following situation: "Sally, what's the *evidence* that you'll never learn all the chemistry?"

4. Do problem-solving with the patient: "Sally, what could you do to learn this material better?"

5. Use the downward arrow technique (see Chapter 10 pp. 145–146) to uncover an underlying belief: "Sally, if it's true that you can't learn all the chemistry, what would that mean to you?"

QUESTIONING TO EVALUATE AN AUTOMATIC THOUGHT

Having elicited an automatic thought, determined that it is important and distressing, and identified its accompanying reactions (emotional, physiological, and behavioral), the therapist may decide to help the patient evaluate it. *He does not directly challenge the automatic thought*, however, for two reasons. First, he does not know in advance that any given automatic thought is distorted. Second, a direct challenge violates a fundamental principal of cognitive therapy, that of collaborative empiricism: The therapist and patient together examine the automatic thought, test its validity and/or utility, and develop a more adaptive response. The therapist keeps in mind that automatic thoughts are rarely completely erroneous. Usually, they contain a grain of truth, and it is important to acknowledge the grain of truth if it exists.

The therapist may use questioning from the very first session to evaluate a specific automatic thought. In the second or third session, he begins to explain the process more explicitly:

T: (*Summarizes past portion of the session; writes automatic thoughts on paper for both to see.*) So when you met your friend, Karen, on the way to the library, you had the thought, "She doesn't really care what happens to me," and that thought made you feel sad?

P: Yeah.

T: And how much did you believe that thought at the time?

P: Oh, pretty much. About 90%.

T: And how sad did you feel?

P: Maybe 80%.

T: Do you remember what we said last week? Sometimes automatic thoughts are true, sometimes they turn out not to be true, and sometimes they have a grain of truth. Can we look at this thought about Karen now and see how accurate it seems?

P: Okay.

T: Here's a list of questions I'd like us to refer to. [See Figure 8.1.] You can keep this copy. We'll look at the first five questions. Let me ask you—what evidence was there that the thought was true, that she didn't really care what happened to you?

P: Well, when we passed on Locust Walk, she seemed like she was real rushed. She just quickly said, "Hi, Sally, see you later," and kept going fast. She hardly even looked at me.

T: Anything else?

P: No . . . nothing I can think of now. Except that sometimes she's pretty busy and doesn't have much time for me.

T: Anything else?

P: No. I guess not.

T: Okay, now is there any evidence on the other side, that maybe she *does* care about what happens to you?

P: (*Answering in general terms.*) Well, she is pretty nice. We've been friends since school started.

T: What kinds of things does she do or say that might show she likes you? (*Helping the patient think more specifically.*)

P: Ummm . . . she usually asks if I want to go get something to eat with her. Sometimes we stay up pretty late just talking about things.

QUESTIONING AUTOMATIC THOUGHTS

1. What is the evidence?
   What is the evidence that supports this idea?
   What is the evidence against this idea?

2. Is there an alternative explanation?

3. What is the *worst* that could happen? Could I live through it?
   What is the best that could happen?
   What is the most realistic outcome?

4. What is the effect of my believing the automatic thought?
   What could be the effect of changing my thinking?

5. What should I do about it?

6. What would I tell _____ (a friend) if he or she were in the same situation?

FIGURE 8.1. Questioning automatic thoughts. Copyright 1993 by Judith S. Beck, Ph.D.

T: Okay. So, on the one hand, on this occasion yesterday, she rushed by you, not saying much. And there have been other times, too, when she's been pretty busy. But, on the other hand, she asks you to eat with her, and you stay up late talking sometimes. Right?

P: Yeah.

The therapist gently probes to *uncover evidence* regarding the validity of Sally's thought. Having elicited evidence on both sides, he summarizes what Sally has already said. In the next section, he helps Sally *devise a reasonable alternative explanation* for what has happened and asks her to *examine possible outcomes*.

T: Good. Now, let's look at the situation again. Could there be another way of explaining what happened, other than she doesn't care about what happens to you?

P: I don't know.

T: Why else might she have rushed by quickly?

P: I'm not sure. She might have had a class. She might have been late for something.

T: Okay. Now, what would be the *worst* that could happen in this situation?

P: That she would truly not like me, I guess. That I couldn't count on her for support.

T: Would you survive that?

P: Yeah. But I wouldn't be happy about it.

T: And what's the *best* that could happen?

P: That she does like me. That she was just rushed then.

T: And what's the *most realistic outcome*?

P: I guess I do think she still likes me.

In the previous section, the therapist helps Sally see that even if the worst happened, she would live through it. Sally also realizes that her worst fears are unlikely to come true. In the next section, Sally's therapist has her *assess the consequences of responding and not responding to her distorted thinking* and then helps her *become problem-solving oriented*, devising a plan to ameliorate this situation.

T: And what is the *effect of your thinking* that she doesn't like you?

P: It makes me sad. I think it kind of makes me withdraw from her.

T: And what could be the *effect of changing your thinking*?

P: I'd feel better.

T: And what do you think you should *do* about this situation?

P: Uh . . . I'm not sure what you mean.

T: Well, have you withdrawn any since this happened yesterday?

P: Yeah, I think so. I didn't say much when I saw her this morning.

T: So this morning you were still acting as if that original thought were true. How could you act differently?

P: I could talk to her more, be friendlier myself.

If Sally's therapist were unsure of Sally's social skills or motivation to carry through with this plan of being friendlier to Karen, he might have spent a few minutes asking Sally such questions as: When might you see her again? Would it be worth it, do you think, to seek her out yourself? What could you say to her when you do see her? Anything you think could get in the way of your saying that? (If needed, he might have modeled for her some things she could say to Karen and/or engaged her in a role-play.)

In the last part of this discussion, Sally's therapist assesses how much Sally now believes the original automatic thought and how she feels emotionally in order to decide what to do next in the session.

T: Good. Now how much do you believe this thought: "Karen doesn't really care what happens to me"?

P: Not very much. Maybe 20%.

T: Okay. And how sad do you feel?

P: Not much either. 20%.

T: Good. It sounds like this exercise was useful. Let's go back and see what we did that helped.

The therapist and patient do not apply all the questions in Figure 8.1 to every automatic thought they evaluate. Sometimes none of the questions seems useful and the therapist takes another tack altogether (see pp. 116–118). The therapist chooses to use the first five questions in this case because his goal for the session is to demonstrate to the patient a structured method to investigate and respond to her thinking. He purposely selects an automatic thought that seems important (i.e., significantly contributes to the patient's distress), is not an isolated idea (but a recurrent theme that is likely to crop up again), seems distorted and dysfunctional, and is likely to serve as a useful model in teaching the patient how to evaluate and respond to other thoughts in the future. He also notes how strongly the patient believes the automatic thought and how intense her emotion is *before and after* the Socratic questioning so he can assess how well this intervention worked.

The therapist may decide to review the process of using Figure 8.1 to confirm that the patient understands how to use it and perceives its value. He might use the same example (as follows) and/or demonstrate with a new example in the next session.

T: Let's review what we just did. We started with an automatic thought, "Karen doesn't really care what happens to me."

P: Right.

T: Then we evaluated that thought using these questions. [See Figure 8.1.] And what happened to your mood?

P: I felt a lot less sad.

T: Do you think evaluating your thoughts with these questions could help you this week if another troublesome situation comes up?

P: It might. But what if a thought turns out to be true?

T: In that case, we would probably do some problem- solving. For example, we might have discussed how you could approach Karen yourself this week. In any case, neither of us knows in advance if evaluating a given thought will be helpful. How do you feel about trying to use these questions sometime this week, when you've iden-tified a thought that has upset you?

P: Okay, sure.

T: If you're like most people, I should warn you, using these questions is sometimes harder than it looks. In fact, there may be times when we really need to work together to help you examine a thought. But give it a try and, if you do have trouble, we can talk about it next week. Okay?

Learning to evaluate automatic thoughts is a skill. Some people grasp it right away; others need much repeated, guided practice. In the previous transcript, the therapist predicts in advance that Sally might have some difficulty because he wants to allay self-criticism or defeatism. Had he suspected, despite his admonition, that Sally would judge herself harshly for not being able to fulfill the homework assignment perfectly, he would have pursued the subject more thoroughly.

T: Sally, if you do have trouble evaluating your thoughts this week, how are you likely to feel?

P: Frustrated, I guess.

T: What's likely to go through your mind?

P: I don't know. I'll probably just quit.

T: Can you imagine looking at the sheet of paper and not being able to figure out what to do?

P: Yeah.

T: What's going through your mind as you look at the paper?

P: "I should be able to do this. I'm so stupid."

T: Good! Now how are you going to answer those thoughts?

The therapist and Sally come up with some coping statements that Sally writes on a card.

Automatic thoughts. *I should be able to do this. I'm so stupid.*

Adaptive response. *Actually, I shouldn't be able to do this. It's a new skill; I'll learn to do it eventually, but it may take more practice with my therapist first. It has nothing to do with whether or not I'm stupid. Either I'm trying to work with a difficult thought or I just need more guidance. In any case, it's no big deal. We predicted this might happen.*

T: Do you think this card will help enough? Or do you think we should put off this assignment until we have more time to practice together?

P: No. I think I can try it.

T: Okay, now if you should get frustrated and have automatic thoughts, be sure to jot them down. Okay?

P: Yeah.

Here the therapist makes the assignment into a no-lose proposition: Either Sally does it successfully or she has some difficulty that the therapist can help her with at the next session. If frustrated, she either reads her card (and probably feels better) or keeps track of her thoughts so she can learn to respond to them in the next session.

Finally, it is important to remember that not all the questions are suitable for every automatic thought. Moreover, using all the questions, even if they all do logically apply, may be too cumbersome and time-consuming. The patient may not evaluate her thoughts at all if she considers the process too burdensome.

T: Okay, so we'll use these questions as a guide this week, but remember not all of them will be relevant. Question 2, especially, often applies in situations where you have a problem with another person, but not in all situations. In the future, you won't necessarily go through this *whole* list of questions, but I'd like you to try them this week to make sure you understand them. In the next couple of weeks, we'll add a couple more. Okay?

Sometimes a patient has difficulty using the questions on the top part of Figure 8.1 because she cannot examine her thought objectively. At these times, it is often useful to have the patient distance herself from the thought in order to evaluate it more rationally. One distancing technique is to have the patient *imagine that the identical situation is happening to a specific friend* and that she is giving the friend advice. The following transcript first demonstrates Sally's difficulty in evaluating a thought and shows how the therapist helps Sally gain a new perspective through the "friend question."

T: Okay, to summarize then, you just got a C– on a surprise quiz, and you had the thought, "I'll never make it [in college]," which made you quite sad.

P: Right.

T: Sally, is there any other evidence that you can't make it?

P: Yeah, I can't seem to concentrate anymore. I just read and read my economics book, and it doesn't get through my head. I have a paper due in 2 weeks, and I haven't started it yet—

T: Any evidence on the other side? That maybe you can make it?

P: No. I don't think so.

At this point, the therapist could help Sally uncover evidence he knows about or guesses might be there: "Didn't you tell me you did better on your first quiz, which was announced? Is that evidence that you can make it? Is it possible that you could have done better if this quiz had been announced? Do you know how everyone else did on this surprise quiz? Are you looking at the grade as if it were an F instead of a C–?" Instead, though, he tries a different tack.

T: Sally, if your roommate were in your situation and had gotten a C– on a surprise economics quiz, and *she* had had the thought, "I'll never make it," what would you tell her?

P: Hmmm . . . I don't know.

T: Would you agree with her? Would you say, "Yeah, Jane, you're probably right, you're not going to make it"?

P: No. Not at all. I guess I'd say, "Listen, this was a surprise quiz, you just weren't ready for it. If you had known about it, you probably would have studied more or gone to see the TA [teaching assistant] for help and you would have done better. It doesn't mean you can't make it. It just took you by surprise."

T: Okay, now how does what you would say to your roommate apply to you?

P: Well, it *was* a surprise. It's true I hadn't studied much for it—I mean I spent an hour staring at the pages, but if I had known there was a quiz, I think I would have made myself concentrate better.

T: Good. So how can you respond to this thought, "I'll never make it," if it comes up again?

In this instance, the therapist supplies a "friend" for Sally to imagine. Usually, though, the therapist asks the patient to supply the name of a specific person: "Sally, I wonder if you can imagine another person in this same situation, maybe a friend or a relative, and imagine they had the same thought."

Having successfully used the technique, the therapist next seeks to maximize the chance that Sally will use it herself, so he explicitly teaches it to her.

T: So was it helpful to evaluate this thought, "I'll never make it," by taking it away from yourself and seeing how you would help your roommate with it, and then seeing how your advice applied to you?

P: Yeah. I guess I could see it more clearly then.

T: Do you have your sheet from last week, the one with questions that help you evaluate automatic thoughts? This question is number 6. If you get a chance this week, how about trying out this question to evaluate an automatic thought? Then if you have any trouble, or you find it's not helpful, we can discuss it next time.

Finally, when the patient has progressed in therapy and can automatically evaluate her thoughts, the therapist may sometimes just ask the patient to *devise an adaptive response*.

P: [When I get ready to ask my roommate to keep the kitchen neater] I'll probably think I should just clean it better myself.

T: Can you think of a more adaptive way to view this?

P: Yeah. That it's better for me to stand up for myself. That I'm doing something reasonable. I'm not being mean or asking her to do more than her share.

T: Good. What do you think will happen to your anxiety if you say that to yourself?

P: It'll go down.

Alternatively, if the therapist judges that a patient's automatic thoughts might interfere with her plans, he might just ask her *how she can respond* (assuming that she is already somewhat proficient at using the aforementioned questions).

T: Anything you can think of that might get in the way of your starting the statistics assignment?

P: I might think there's too much to do and get overwhelmed.

T: Okay, if you do have the thought, "There's too much to do," what can you tell yourself?

P: That I don't have to do it all in one night, that I don't have to understand it perfectly this first time through.

T: Good. Will that be enough, do you think, to go ahead and start the assignment?

USING ALTERNATIVE QUESTIONING

The beginning cognitive therapist is advised to use Figure 8.1 as a guide when initially evaluating automatic thoughts. These standard questions, however, frequently need to be modified for specific automatic thoughts. Various examples of different types of Socratic questions are described by Overholser (1993a, 1993b).

The following transcript is just one illustration of how the therapist varies his questioning when he judges that the standard questions will be ineffective.

T: What went through your mind [when you asked your mom if it was all right with her to shorten your time together and she sounded hurt and angry]?

P: That I should have known it was a bad time to call. I shouldn't have called.

T: What's the evidence that you shouldn't have called?

P: Well, my mother is usually rushed in the morning. If I had waited until after she got home from work, she might have been in a better frame of mind.

T: Had that occurred to you?

P: Well, yeah, but I wanted to let my roommate know right away if I could visit her or not so she could make plans.

T: So you actually had a reason for calling when you did, and it sounds as if you knew it might be risky but you really wanted to let your roommate know as soon as you could?

P: Yeah.

T: Is it reasonable to be so hard on yourself for taking the risk?

P: No—

T: You don't sound convinced. How bad is it anyway, in the scheme of things, for your mom to feel hurt that you want to spend part of your summer vacation with your roommate?

The therapist follows up these questions with others: How hurt did your mother feel? How long did the hurt last at that level? How does she probably feel now? Is it possible for you to spare your mother hurt all the time? Can you possibly do what is good for you and not hurt your mother at all—given that she wants to spend as much time with you as she can? Is it desirable to have a goal of *never* hurting someone else's feelings? What would you have to give up yourself?

T: Let's go back to the original thoughts, "I should have known it was a bad time to call. I should have waited." How do you see it now?

P: Well, it wasn't such a terrible thing. She probably would have felt somewhat hurt no matter when I called because she does want to spend as much time with me as she can. But maybe that's not good for me, always doing what she wants and ignoring what's good for me. I guess she'll get over it.

The previous transcript demonstrates how the therapist varies his questioning to help the patient adopt a more functional perspective. Although he starts out questioning the *validity* of the thought, he shifts the emphasis to the *implicit underlying belief* (which they had previously discussed in other contexts): It is bad to hurt other people's feelings. At the end, he asks Sally an open-ended question ("How do you see the situation now?") to assess the effect of the questioning and to evaluate whether further work on the automatic thought is required. Note that many questions the therapist asked were a variation of question 2 in Figure 8.1: Is there an alternative explanation (for why you called when you did and for why your mother was hurt [other than that you were bad and at fault])?

IDENTIFYING COGNITIVE DISTORTIONS

Patients tend to make consistent errors in their thinking. Often there is a systematic negative bias in the cognitive processing of patients who suffer from a psychiatric disorder (Beck, 1976). When the patient expresses an automatic thought, the therapist notes (mentally, verbally, or in writing) the type of error she seems to be making. The most common errors are presented in Figure 8.2 (see also Burns, 1980).

Some patients like the intellectual challenge of labeling their distortions themselves. The therapist might give this type of patient a copy of Figure 8.2.

T: We've been talking about how when people are distressed they often have thoughts which are not true or not wholly true. Right?

P: Right.

T: I have a list here to give you that describes the most common mistakes people make in their thinking. Often it's helpful to try to figure out what mistake you might be making because it'll help you respond to the thought better. Let me show you the list so you can see if you'd like to try to use it.

P: Okay.

T: So here are 12 common mistakes. Let's see if we can identify any you've made recently. The first one is "all-or-nothing thinking" where you see things in very black and white terms, instead of shades of gray. . . . How about when you had the thought last week, "Either I get an A or I'm a failure"? Can you see how that's very black and white?

P: Yeah.

T: Can you think of any other examples? [The therapist and patient spend another couple of minutes on this cognitive distortion. Then the therapist picks another distortion typical of this patient, and they review this second kind of error in the same way.] Anyway, for homework would you like to label the distortion when you catch an automatic thought? We can keep this sheet in front of us during our sessions, too, and occasionally see if we can figure out the distortion when we talk about other automatic thoughts.

For many patients, the list in Figure 8.2 is overwhelming. In this case, the therapist might label and describe just the distortions typical of this patient:

Although some automatic thoughts are true, many are either untrue or have just a grain of truth. Typical mistakes in thinking include:

1. *All-or-nothing thinking* (also called black-and-white, polarized, or dichotomous thinking): You view a situation in only two categories instead of on a continuum.
   Example: "If I'm not a total success, I'm a failure."
2. *Catastrophizing* (also called fortune telling): You predict the future negatively without considering other, more likely outcomes.
   Example: "I'll be so upset, I won't be able to function at all."
3. *Disqualifying or discounting the positive*: You unreasonably tell yourself that positive experiences, deeds, or qualities do not count.
   Example: "I did that project well, but that doesn't mean I'm competent; I just got lucky."
4. *Emotional reasoning*: You think something must be true because you "feel" (actually believe) it so strongly, ignoring or discounting evidence to the contrary.
   Example: "I know I do a lot of things okay at work, but I still feel like I'm a failure."
5. *Labeling*: You put a fixed, global label on yourself or others without considering that the evidence might more reasonably lead to a less disastrous conclusion.
   Example: "I'm a loser. He's no good."
6. *Magnification/minimization*: When you evaluate yourself, another person, or a situation, you unreasonably magnify the negative and/or minimize the positive.
   Example: "Getting a mediocre evaluation proves how inadequate I am. Getting high marks doesn't mean I'm smart."
7. *Mental filter* (also called selective abstraction): You pay undue attention to one negative detail instead of seeing the whole picture.
   Example: "Because I got one low rating on my evaluation [which also contained several high ratings] it means I'm doing a lousy job."
8. *Mind reading*: You believe you know what others are thinking, failing to consider other, more likely possibilities.
   Example: "He's thinking that I don't know the first thing about this project."
9. *Overgeneralization*: You make a sweeping negative conclusion that goes far beyond the current situation.
   Example: "[Because I felt uncomfortable at the meeting] I don't have what it takes to make friends."
10. *Personalization*: You believe others are behaving negatively because of you, without considering more plausible explanations for their behavior.
    Example: "The repairman was curt to me because I did something wrong."
11. *"Should" and "must" statements* (also called imperatives): You have a precise, fixed idea of how you or others should behave and you overestimate how bad it is that these expectations are not met.
    Example: "It's terrible that I made a mistake. I should always do my best."
12. *Tunnel vision*: You only see the negative aspects of a situation.
    Example: "My son's teacher can't do anything right. He's critical and insensitive and lousy at teaching."

FIGURE 8.2. Thinking errors. Adapted with permission from Aaron T. Beck, M.D.

T: Well, we've just identified a number of automatic thoughts you had this week about your job, your health, and your children. I wonder if you see a common thread—in each case, it seems that you're predicting the worst that could happen. Is that right?

P: Yeah.

T: When people predict the worst, we call it fortune telling or catastrophizing—believing that a catastrophe might happen. Are you aware of catastrophizing much?

P: I think I probably do.

T: How about if you try this week to catch yourself catastrophizing? When you write down an automatic thought, see if that's what you're doing, and if so, write "catastrophizing" next to it.

A third option is to offer the list of distortions to the patient but to check off only one, two, or three errors most common to that patient so she does not become overwhelmed by trying to focus on them all. When the patient can determine the type of distortion she is making, she can often evaluate the validity of her thought more objectively. The next section describes how to help patients assess how *useful* their thoughts are.

QUESTIONING TO EVALUATE THE UTILITY OF AUTOMATIC THOUGHTS

Some automatic thoughts may be entirely valid or, despite evaluation, a patient may still believe they are entirely valid when they are not. At these times, the *usefulness* of the thought is assessed. The therapist can either help the patient determine the effect of her thinking (as in question 4 from Figure 8.1) or ask specifically for the advantages and disadvantages of continuing to have the thought, followed by an adaptive response to the thought.

T: Sally, you may be right that your chances aren't good to get the summer job you want. But what's the advantage of continuously telling yourself, "I'll never get it, I'll never get it"?

P: Well, I won't be so disappointed when I don't.

T: And what's the disadvantage of saying it over and over?

P: The disadvantage?

T: Does that thought bring you great satisfaction? Does it help you get your application finished? Does it enhance your enjoyment of school?

P: No.

T: So you can see that saying you'll never get it has disadvantages?

P: Yeah.

T: What would be a useful response, then, when you have the thought, "I'll never get the job"?

P: I will get the job?

T: Well, I wonder if that might be taking *too* rosy a view. How about reminding yourself of the likelihood that you will get *some* job, even if it's not your first choice. Then maybe you could remind yourself to refocus your attention on whatever you're doing. Do you think that could help? . . . Do you want to try that this week?

At another time the therapist might turn his attention to the thought, "I'll never get the job I want," and explore the underlying meaning. In this session, however, he chooses to explore the utility of the automatic thought. In the next section, he explicitly teaches the process to the patient.

T: Sally, let's review what we just did. We started with the thought, "I'll never get the summer job I want." We looked at the evidence that the thought is true, but it turned out that it isn't all that clear whether your prediction is probably right or not. So then we looked at how *useful* the thought is. Do you remember how we judged that?

P: Yeah. We looked at the advantages and disadvantages.

T: Right. And discovering it was pretty disadvantageous, we came up with a plan of how to respond to that thought the next time it comes up. So even when a thought is true, or when you truly can't evaluate it, you can still respond to it, based on its disadvantages.

ASSESSING THE EFFECTIVENESS OF EVALUATING THE AUTOMATIC THOUGHT

Having used standard or nonstandard questions (or a behavioral experiment; see Chapter 12, pp. 197–200) to evaluate an automatic thought, the therapist assesses the effectiveness of the evaluation in order to decide what to do next in the session. If the patient no longer believes the automatic thought as much and if her emotional reaction has decreased significantly, the therapist has an indication that he should move on to something else.

T: How much do you believe now that Jane will get angry and stay angry with you if you bring up the problem of noise?

P: Not much. Maybe 25%.

T: And how worried do you feel now?

P: Less. About 20%.

T: Good. Anything else on this? No? How about if we move on to the next thing on the agenda.

CONCEPTUALIZING WHY THE EVALUATION OF AN AUTOMATIC THOUGHT WAS INEFFECTIVE

If the patient still believes the automatic thought to a significant degree and does not feel better emotionally, the therapist seeks to understand why this initial attempt at cognitive restructuring has not been sufficiently effective. Common reasons to consider include the following:

1. There are other more central automatic thoughts and/or images left unidentified or unevaluated.
2. The evaluation of the automatic thought is implausible, superficial, or inadequate.
3. The patient has not sufficiently expressed the evidence she believes supports the automatic thought.
4. The automatic thought itself is also a core belief.
5. The patient understands "intellectually" that the automatic thought is distorted but does not believe it on a more "emotional" level.
6. The patient discounts the evaluation.

In the first situation, *the therapist has not elicited the most central automatic thought or image.* Sally, for example, reports the thought, "If I try out [for the school newspaper], I probably won't make it." Evaluating this thought does not significantly affect her dysphoria because she has other important (but unrecognized) thoughts: "What if they [the editors] think I'm a lousy writer?" "What if I write something really bad?" She also has an image of the editors reading her article with mocking, scornful faces.

In a second situation, *the patient responds to an automatic thought superficially*. Sally has the thought, "I won't finish all my work. I have too much to do." Instead of carefully evaluating the thought, Sally merely responds, "No, I'll probably get it done." This response is insufficient, and Sally's anxiety does not decrease.

In a third situation, *the therapist does not sufficiently elicit the patient's evidence that her automatic thought is true*, resulting in an ineffective adaptive response, as seen here:

T: Okay, Sally, what evidence do you have that your brother doesn't want to bother with you?

P: Well, he hardly ever calls me. I always call him.

T: Okay, anything on the other side? That he does care about you, that he does want a good relationship with you?

Had Sally's therapist probed a little more, he would have uncovered other evidence that Sally has to support her automatic thought: that her brother spent more time with his girlfriend during vacations than with Sally, that he sounded impatient on the phone whenever she called, and that he had not sent her a birthday card. Having elicited this additional data, the therapist could have helped Sally weigh the evidence more effectively and investigated alternative explanations for her brother's behavior.

In a fourth situation, *the patient identifies an automatic thought that is also a core belief*. Sally often has the thought, "I'm incompetent." She believes this idea so strongly that a single evaluation does not alter her perception or the associated affect. Her therapist needs to use many techniques over time to alter this belief (see Chapter 11).

In a fifth situation, *the patient indicates that she believes an adaptive response "intellectually," in her mind, but not "emotionally," in her heart, soul, or gut*. In this case, the therapist and patient need to explore an unarticulated belief that lies *behind* the automatic thought.

T: How much do you believe that the professor won't think you're wasting his time and, even if he does, that's his job?

P: Well, I can see it intellectually.

T: But?

P: Even though I think he should help me, I still think he'll think I'm wasting his time.

T: Okay, let's assume for a moment that he *does* think you're wasting his time, what's so bad about that?

Here, Sally's therapist discovers that she does not really believe the adaptive response and uncovers an underlying belief: If I ask for help, it means I am weak.

In a sixth situation, the patient discounts the adaptive response.

T: How much do you believe that the professor won't think you're wasting his time or, if he does, that that's what he's being paid for anyway?

P: I do believe it, but—

T: But?

P: But I still think I should work it out myself.

T: Well, that's another possibility, maybe you should. Should we look rationally at whether you're better off working it out yourself or going to him for help?

P: Okay.

Discounting the adaptive response often takes the form of a "yes, but . . . " statement: "Yes, I believe [this response], but . . . . " The "yes, but . . . " statement can then be treated as another automatic thought and subjected to rational evaluation.

To summarize, having evaluated an automatic thought, the therapist asks the patient to rate how much she believes the adaptive response and how she feels emotionally. If her belief is low, and she is still distressed, he tries to conceptualize why the examination of the thought did not alleviate her distress. The next chapter describes how to help patients respond to their automatic thoughts.

Chapter 9

RESPONDING TO AUTOMATIC THOUGHTS

The previous chapter demonstrated the use of questioning to help a patient evaluate an automatic thought and determine the effectiveness of the evaluation. In many cases the therapist chooses to follow up this verbal interaction with another intervention to fortify a more adaptive viewpoint. This follow-up activity is often a written response which the patient can read for homework. Writing down important learnings during the therapy session not only reinforces new understandings at the time but also provides an opportunity for the patient to refer to important therapy notes weeks and months (and even years) after therapy has ended. This chapter describes the Dysfunctional Thought Record, the primary tool for patients to evaluate and respond in writing to their automatic thoughts, and other methods for responding to automatic thoughts.

DYSFUNCTIONAL THOUGHT RECORDS

The Dysfunctional Thought Record (DTR), also known in an earlier version as the Daily Record of Dysfunctional Thoughts (Beck et al., 1979), is a worksheet that helps a patient respond more effectively to her automatic thoughts, thereby reducing her dysphoria (see Figure 9.1). Some patients use it quite consistently. Others, despite the best efforts of their therapist, cannot or will not write down their thoughts and so rarely use it. Most patients fall someplace in the middle; that is, with proper instruction and encouragement from the therapist, they use DTRs on a fairly regular basis. If the therapist judges that a patient may be overwhelmed by the format of the DTR, he may teach the patient to use the questions listed in Chapter 8, Figure 8.1, instead.

Directions: When you notice your mood getting worse, ask yourself, "What's going through my mind right now?" and as soon as possible jot down the thought or mental image in the Automatic Thought column.

Date/time	Situation	Automatic thought(s)	Emotion(s)	Adaptive response	Outcome
	1. What actual event or stream of thoughts, or daydreams or recollection led to the unpleasant emotion? 2. What (if any) distressing physical sensations did you have?	1. What thought(s) and/or image(s) went through your mind? 2. How much did you believe each one at the time?	1. What emotion(s) (sad/anxious/ angry/etc.) did you feel at the time? 2. How intense (0–100%) was the emotion?	1. (optional) What cognitive distortion did you make? 2. Use questions at bottom to compose a response to the automatic thought(s). 3. How much do you believe each response?	1. How much do you now believe each automatic thought? 2. What emotion(s) do you feel now? How intense (0–100%) is the emotion? 3. What will you do (or did you do)?
Friday 2/23 10 A.M.	Talking on the phone with Donna.	She must not like me any more. 90%	Sad 80%		
Tuesday 2/27 12 P.M.	Studying for my exam.	I'll never learn this. 100%	Sad 95%		
Thursday 2/29 5 P.M.	Thinking about my economics class tomorrow.	I might get called on and I won't give a good answer. 80%	Anxious 80%		
	Noticing my heart beating fast and my trouble concentrating.	What's wrong with me?	Anxious 80%		

Questions to help compose an alternative response: (1) What is the evidence that the automatic thought is true? Not true? (2) Is there an alternative explanation? (3) What's the worst that could happen? Could I live through it? What's the best that could happen? What's the most realistic outcome? (4) What's the effect of my believing the automatic thought? What could be the effect of my changing my thinking? (5) What should I do about it? (6) If _____ [friend's name] was in the situation and had this thought, what would I tell him/her?

FIGURE 9.1. Dysfunctional thought record. Copyright 1995 by Judith S. Beck, Ph.D.

126

Patients are more likely to use the DTR if it is properly introduced, demonstrated, and practiced. A few guidelines are suggested:

1. The therapist should have mastered the DTR himself (with his own automatic thoughts) before presenting it to a patient.

2. The therapist should plan to introduce the DTR in two stages over two or more sessions. Stage 1 covers the first four columns; Stage 2, the last two columns.

3. The therapist should ascertain that the patient really grasps and believes in the cognitive model before introducing the DTR (otherwise she will not understand the value of identifying and evaluating her thoughts).

4. The patient should demonstrate an ability to identify her automatic thoughts and emotions before being introduced to the DTR. She should be able to state the situation, her emotions, and her physiological response without confusing these three with automatic thoughts. If she does not have a clear understanding and ability to differentiate among these phenomena, she will most likely experience difficulty with the DTR. Thus, the therapist should verbally elicit several clear, important examples of specific situations with their accompanying automatic thoughts and emotions prior to demonstrating how to record such data on a DTR.

5. The patient should demonstrate success in completing the first four columns on her own with several different situations before being introduced to the last two columns.

6. The therapist should have *verbally* evaluated at least one important automatic thought with a patient and have produced some decrease in dysphoria prior to demonstrating how to complete the last two columns.

7. If the patient fails to complete homework assignments using the DTR, the therapist should elicit automatic thoughts about doing the DTR itself, help with practical problem-solving, propose doing a DTR as an experiment, consider disclosing his own use of the DTR, and otherwise motivate the patient.

Having identified a problematic situation, the therapist first helps the patient identify specific automatic thoughts and the associated emotions through verbal questioning alone. He may choose these examples to illustrate the use of the DTR. If the therapist presents the DTR without first successfully identifying an important situation, automatic thought, and emotion, he runs the risk of confusing the patient if she subsequently cannot correctly identify these different items.

In the following section, the therapist has already ascertained the content of the first four columns of the DTR for a specific automatic thought before he presents the patient with a blank DTR.

THERAPIST: Okay, Sally, let me make sure I understand. The situation was that your high school friend Donna called and said she couldn't come this weekend. You had the thought, "She must not like me anymore," and you felt sad. Is that right?

PATIENT: Yes.

T: Good. Now in a few minutes I'd like us to evaluate that thought, but first I'd like to show you a worksheet that I think will help you. It's called a DTR—a Dysfunctional Thought Record—and it's just an organized way of responding to thoughts that are distressing you. Okay? (*Pulls out Figure 9.1.*)

P: Sure.

T: Here it is. Today we'll concentrate on the first four columns, so I'll just cross out the last two. We'll look at them at another session. Now, before I start, I have to tell you a couple of things. First, spelling, handwriting, and grammar don't count.

P: (*Laughs.*)

T: Second, this is a useful tool, and it may take some practice for you to get really good at it. So expect to make some mistakes along the way. These mistakes will actually be useful—we'll see what was confusing so you can do it better the next time. Okay?

P: Uh huh.

T: Okay. How about if we use your thought, "She must not like me any more," as an example. The first column is easy. When did you have that thought?

P: Today. This morning.

T: Okay. In the first column put down today's date and about what time it was.

P: (*Does so.*)

T: Would you put down the day of the week, too? I think it'll make it easier for us when we refer back to it. Now, in this second column, you write down the situation. When you had the thought, "She must not like me any more," were you on the phone with her, or did you have it afterwards?

P: It was while I was talking to her.

T: Okay. Under situation, you could write, "Talking on the phone with Donna." If you had had the thought later, you could have written, "Thinking about my phone call with Donna." So the situation can either be an *actual* event or what you're *thinking* about or imagining in your mind. Is that clear?

P: I think so.

T: We'll be going over a lot of examples so it'll become clearer to you. You'll see, too, that the questions at the top of the column prompt you. There's a third kind of situation, too, if your automatic thought is about how you're feeling, emotionally or physically. For example, the situation might be "Noticing that I feel sad," and the thought might be, "I shouldn't be feeling this way. I'm hopeless."

P: Okay. I think I get it.

T: Now, the next column is for the automatic thoughts. Here's where you write down the actual words or pictures that went through your mind. In this case, you had the thought, "She must not like me any more." . . . How much did you believe the thought at that time?

P: A lot: 90%.

T: Good. Write down the thought and then write 90% next to it. . . . And in the fourth column, you write your emotion and how intense it was. In this case, how sad did you feel?

P: Pretty sad: 80%.

T: Okay, write that down. How about if we try this again. Do you remember another time this week when you noticed your mood changing?

P: Sure . . . I was looking for a book at the library today. I started feeling really sad.

T: Okay, let's go back to that time. It's earlier today, you're at the library, looking for a book. You start feeling really sad and now you ask yourself the question at the top of the DTR: *"What is going through my mind right now?" (Circles or highlights this question on the DTR.)*

P: I'll never make it here. I can't even find the book I need.

T: Okay, let's see if you can fill in the first four columns of the DTR yourself. I'll help if need be.

When the patient has successfully completed the first four columns in session with little or no assistance, the therapist may collaboratively set a follow-up homework assignment.

T: Okay, Sally, how would you feel about trying to fill in the first four columns a few times this week for homework? You'll use a change in your mood as a cue to pull this out and ask yourself what's going through your mind, just as it says at the top here.

P: Okay.

T: Let me remind you of a couple of things. First, you don't have to fill it out in order from left to right. Sometimes it's easier to identify the emotion you're feeling first—sad, anxious, angry, and so on—and write it down before you figure out the automatic thought you've just had. Also, you'll remember that this is a skill, and you may not do it perfectly the first time you try it, right? But the more you practice it, the better you'll become at it and the more helpful it can be.

P: Okay.

T: Do you think you could try to write down one automatic thought a day this week?

P: Sure. I'll try.

In the next session, the therapist realizes that Sally has some confusion about situations and automatic thoughts, physiological responses, and emotions (see bottom of Figure 9.1), so he postpones the introduction of the last two columns and instead reviews the DTR that Sally did for homework.

T: Okay, let's take a look at this DTR you did at home. This first example looks good. On Tuesday, you were studying for an exam; you had the thought, "I'll never learn this," which you believed 100%; and you felt 95% sad. Good. If we have time today, we'll evaluate that thought, but first let's talk about this second item you wrote down.

P: I didn't do it right. I couldn't figure out what my automatic thought was.

T: Okay, let's look at it. I see it was yesterday, around 5:00. What were you doing?

P: Well, I should have been studying, but I couldn't, like concentrate very well. I was walking around my room—

T: What were you thinking about?

P: About my economics class that I had today. I thought I might get called on and I was sure I wouldn't give a good answer.

T: Oh, so you had the thought, "I might get called on and I won't give a good answer."

P: Yeah.

T: Good. Write that under "automatic thought." . . . Now at the time, how much did you believe this thought?

P: About 80%.

T: Okay. Write that down. . . . Now how did that thought make you feel?

P: Anxious. My heart started beating fast.

T: How anxious, 0–100%?

P: About 80%.

T: Write that down under emotion: anxious, 80%. Now under situation, write down, "Thinking about class tomorrow." . . . Okay, it sounds like "heart beating fast" and "difficulty concentrating" were symptoms of anxiety. Did anything go through your mind about these symptoms?

P: Yeah. I was thinking, "What's wrong with me?"

T: Okay. So a second situation was noticing your heart beating fast and having trouble concentrating; and the automatic thought was, "What's wrong with me?" Can you fill those things in, too?

At the next session, her therapist notes that Sally has mastered the first four columns of the DTR, as evidenced by her homework. One of his goals for the session, if the opportunity arises, is to teach Sally to use the last two columns. He uses the questions at the bottom of the DTR to help her evaluate one of the thoughts she had written down for homework (see Figure 9.2). He does so verbally at first, to make sure the use of these questions is effective.

T: Okay, now let's see if you can transfer some of what we just talked about to the DTR. What cognitive distortion did we say you made?

P: Fortune telling.

T: Okay, you can write that at the top of fourth column, which is called "adaptive response." Do you see the instructions for this column? Writing down the type of cognitive distortion is optional.

P: Okay.

T: Next, you use the questions at the bottom of the DTR to evaluate your thinking and compose an adaptive response in column 4. These questions are the same ones we used just a minute ago when we did this verbally.

P: Okay.

T: First we looked at the evidence, and what did you conclude?

P: That I don't really know if Bob wants to go out or not. That he does act friendly to me in class.

T: Okay, write down those two things in the fifth column. . . . Now, how much do you believe each statement?

P: Oh, pretty much: 90%.

Directions: When you notice your mood getting worse, ask yourself, "What's going through my mind right now?" and as soon as possible jot down the thought or mental image in the Automatic Thought column.

Date/time	Situation	Automatic thought(s)	Emotion(s)	Adaptive response	Outcome
	1. What actual event or stream of thoughts, or daydreams or recollection led to the unpleasant emotion? 2. What (if any) distressing physical sensations did you have?	1. What thought(s) and/or image(s) went through your mind? 2. How much did you believe each one at the time?	1. What emotion(s) (sad/anxious/angry /etc.) did you feel at the time? 2. How intense (0–100%) was the emotion?	1. (optional) What cognitive distortion did you make? 2. Use questions at bottom to compose a response to the automatic thought(s). 3. How much do you believe each response?	1. How much do you now believe each automatic thought? 2. What emotion(s) do you feel now? How intense (0–100%) is the emotion? 3. What will you do (or did you do)?
Friday 3/8 3 P.M.	Thinking about asking Bob if he wants to have coffee.	He won't want to go with me. 90%	Sad 75%	(Fortune-telling error) I don't really know if he wants to or not. (90%) He is friendly to me in class. (90%) The worst that'll happen is he'll say no and I'll feel bad for a while. (90%) The best is he'll say yes. (100%) The most realistic is he may say he's busy but still act friendly. (80%) If I keep on assuming he doesn't want to go out with me, I'll have no chance with him. (100%) I should just go up and ask him. (50%) What's the big deal, anyway. (75%)	1. AT—50% 2. Sad—50% Anxious—50%

Questions to help compose an alternative response: (1) What is the evidence that the automatic thought is true? Not true? (2) Is there an alternative explanation? (3) What's the worst that could happen? Could I live through it? What's the best that could happen? What's the most realistic outcome? (4) What's the effect of my believing the automatic thought? What could be the effect of my changing my thinking? (5) What should I do about it? (6) If _____ [friend's name] was in the situation and had this thought,, what would I tell him/her?

FIGURE 9.2. Dysfunctional Thought Record. Copyright 1995 by Judith S. Beck, Ph.D.

T: Good. Put 90% next to each statement. . . . Next, we looked at the consequences. What's the best, worst, and most realistic outcome? (*The patient continues to write down the adaptive response and her degree of belief in each statement.*) Good. Now let's look at the last column. How much do you believe your automatic thought now?

P: Maybe 50%.

T: And how do you feel now?

P: Not quite so sad. But more anxious.

T: Okay, in the last column, write down "A.T." for automatic thought and next to it, 50%. Then write down "sad" and rate the degree of sadness 0–100%.

P: (*Does so.*)

T: Now, maybe we should look at the thought that's making you anxious.

Next, the therapist might have the patient practice the DTR with another automatic thought, set a homework assignment using the DTR, or proceed to another topic.

MOTIVATING PATIENTS TO USE DYSFUNCTIONAL THOUGHT RECORDS

Some patients immediately gravitate to the Dysfunctional Thought Record and consistently use it when they feel upset. For others, the following interchange may help:

T: Well, Sally, it looks as if this DTR [the one they just did together] has helped. Your sadness went from 75% down to 50%.

P: Yeah.

T: Do you think using this form could help in the future?

P: Yeah.

T: You're already pretty good at evaluating and answering back your thoughts in your head. But most people find it's much more effective to put it down on paper. What do you think?

P: I think it would help.

T: How likely are you to try it at home this week?

P: I guess I could try it.

T: You know, I occasionally still do DTRs myself when I find I'm overreacting. I find it's much more helpful to do it on paper than just doing it mentally. But we don't really know if that's true for you. How would you feel about doing an experiment? At least once this week, you could adaptively respond to your thoughts in your head. See how it affects your mood. Then pull out the DTR and put it all on paper and see if you feel even better. What do you think?

P: Okay.

T: How likely is it that you'll try this experiment?

P: I will.

In order to encourage the patient to try the DTR, the therapist asks the patient to try an experiment. If she returns the following week with a correctly completed thought record (which has been effective in modifying her mood), she may not need further motivation. If she did not complete a DTR, did not do it correctly, or did not experience an improvement in mood, the therapist will try to determine why difficulties arose and plan accordingly. At times, commonsense suggestions smooth the way:

P: I know I'll probably have a lot of automatic thoughts during class. But I can't write a DTR then and there.

T: That's true. Do you think it might help to predict a typical, upsetting thought in advance and write a DTR *before* class? Or maybe you could just jot down the automatic thoughts on a piece of paper during class and transfer them to a DTR afterwards.

P: Well, it probably would help to do one beforehand so maybe I won't start off so anxious, but unless I'm coming from therapy, I won't have one with me.

T: Some people carry a blank DTR in their wallet. Would that work for you?

P: Yeah. I guess the only problem would be *where* to write it. I wouldn't want anyone else to see it.

T: Sometimes you have to be inventive. Some people do it at their desk like any other paperwork, or in the car, or even in the bathroom. How about if you see what you can come up with? If you have trouble or if you're still concerned about other people seeing it, we can talk more about it next week.

A discussion of the patient's concerns in the following session might involve identification of automatic thoughts and images about others seeing the DTR, about hopelessness related to being able to feel better, about not wanting to put forth the effort required to modify her mood, or other dysfunctional ideas which get in the way of the patient doing the DTR.

WHEN THE DYSFUNCTIONAL THOUGHT RECORD IS NOT SUFFICIENTLY HELPFUL

As with any technique in cognitive therapy, it is important not to overemphasize its importance. Most patients, at some point, find that completing a particular DTR did not provide much relief. By emphasizing its *general* usefulness and "stuck points" as an opportunity for learning, the therapist helps the patient avoid automatic thoughts critical of herself, the therapy, the therapist, or the DTR itself.

Depending on the individual patient, the therapist might explain common reasons why a DTR did not significantly reduce the patient's dysphoria. As described in the previous chapter, evaluation of an automatic thought (with or without a DTR) may be less than optimally effective if the patient failed to respond to her most upsetting thought or image, if her automatic thought was a core belief or activated an underlying belief, if her evaluation and response were superficial, or if she discounted her response.

ADDITIONAL WAYS TO RESPOND TO AUTOMATIC THOUGHTS

This chapter has thus far emphasized written methods to respond to automatic thoughts. It is not practical or desirable, however, for a patient to respond to every automatic thought in writing. If she did so, her life would become consumed with such an undertaking. In fact, some patients (especially those with obsessive–compulsive personality disorder) may use the DTR too much. Other patients cannot or will not do written assignments. The following are alternative techniques which do not require writing.

1. Doing a DTR mentally.
2. Reading a previously written DTR or notes from therapy that contain an identical or similar automatic thought.
3. Dictating a modified version of a DTR to someone else to write down or having someone else read previously written responses (if the patient can understand but cannot read or write herself).
4. Reading a coping card (see Chapter 12, pp. 214–216).
5. Listening to a therapy session or part of one on audiotape.

Finally, it is more useful at times to do problem-solving instead of evaluating an automatic thought. Sally, for example, had the thought, "I'll never learn the econ stuff before the test." Through careful questioning, her therapist concluded that if Sally continued studying as she had been, it was indeed likely that she *would not* learn the material adequately. He judged that it would be a better use of therapy time to help her devise possible solutions to her real-life problems, including borrowing notes from a classmate, going to the professor for help, outlining the textbook chapters as she read, arranging to study with a friend, and so on.

In summary, the therapist teaches the patient a variety of ways to respond to her distorted thinking. Careful teaching of the DTR maximizes the chance that patients will use this important tool themselves, but there are also other ways for patients to respond to their automatic thoughts if they cannot or will not use a DTR.

Chapter 10

IDENTIFYING AND MODIFYING INTERMEDIATE BELIEFS

Previous chapters described the identification and modification of automatic thoughts, the actual words or images that go through a patient's mind in a given situation and lead to distress. This chapter describes the deeper, often unarticulated ideas or understandings that patients have about themselves, others, and their personal worlds which give rise to specific automatic thoughts. These ideas are often not expressed before therapy but can easily be elicited from the patient or inferred and then tested.

As described in Chapter 2, these beliefs may be classified into two categories: intermediate beliefs (composed of rules, attitudes, and assumptions) and core beliefs (absolutistic, rigid, global ideas about oneself and/or others). Intermediate beliefs, while not as easily modifiable as automatic thoughts, are still more malleable than core belief(s).

This chapter is divided into two parts. In the first part, *cognitive conceptualization* (initially introduced in Chapter 2) is described, and the process of developing a Cognitive Conceptualization Diagram is illustrated. Conceptualization is emphasized throughout this volume to help the therapist plan therapy, become adept at choosing appropriate interventions, and overcome "stuck" points when standard interventions fail. *Eliciting and modifying intermediate beliefs* are the focus of the second part of this chapter. These techniques are also applicable to the next chapter, which presents additional specialized techniques for eliciting and modifying core beliefs.

COGNITIVE CONCEPTUALIZATION

Generally, a therapist and patient work on automatic thoughts first before tackling beliefs. From the beginning, though, the therapist starts formulating a conceptualization, which logically connects automatic thoughts to the deeper-level beliefs. If the therapist fails to see this larger picture, he will be less likely to direct therapy in an effective, efficient way. Novice cognitive therapists often jump from one intermediate belief to another instead of identifying the most central beliefs and doing sustained work on them.

Therefore, the therapist should start filling in a Cognitive Conceptualization Diagram (Figure 10.1) as soon as he has gathered data about the patient's typical automatic thoughts, emotions, behavior, and/or beliefs. This diagram depicts, among other things, the relationship between core beliefs, intermediate beliefs, and current automatic thoughts. It provides a cognitive map of the patient's psychopathology and helps organize the multitude of data that the patient presents. The diagram in Figure 10.1 illustrates the basic questions the therapist asks himself in order to complete the diagram.

Initially, the therapist may have data to complete only a portion of the diagram. He either leaves blank other boxes or fills in items he has inferred with a question mark to indicate their tentative status. He checks out with the patient missing or inferred items at future sessions. The therapist at some point shares the conceptualization with the patient, when his goal for a session is to help the patient understand the broader picture of her difficulties. At that time, he reviews the conceptualization orally, develops a fresh diagram with the patient, or presents the completed diagram. Whenever the therapist presents his interpretations, he labels them as hypotheses, asking the patient whether they "ring true" to her. Correct hypotheses generally resonate with the patient.

Usually it is best to start with the bottom half of the conceptualization diagram. The therapist jots down three *typical* situations in which the patient became upset. Then, for each situation, he fills in the key automatic thought, its meaning, and the patient's subsequent emotion and relevant behavior (if any). If he has not directly asked the patient for the meaning of her automatic thoughts, he either hypothesizes (with a written question mark) or, better still, does the downward arrow technique (pp. 145–146) with the patient at the next session to uncover the meaning for each thought.

The meaning of the automatic thought for each situation should be logically connected with the Core Belief box near the top of the diagram. For example, Sally's diagram (Figure 10.2) clearly shows how her automatic thoughts and the meaning of those thoughts are related to her core belief of inadequacy.

COGNITIVE CONCEPTUALIZATION DIAGRAM

Patient's name:_____**Date:**_____

Diagnosis: Axis I _____**Axis II** _____

Relevant Childhood Data

Which experiences contributed to the development and maintenance of the core belief?

Core Belief(s)

What is the most central belief about herself?

Conditional Assumptions/Beliefs/Rules

Which positive assumption helped her cope with the core belief?

What is the negative counterpart to this assumption?

Compensatory Strategy(ies)

Which behaviors help her cope with the belief?

Situation 1	**Situation 2**	**Situation 3**
What was the problematic situation?		
Automatic Thought	**Automatic Thought**	**Automatic Thought**
What went through her mind?		
Meaning of the A.T.	**Meaning of the A.T.**	**Meaning of the A.T.**
What did the automatic thought mean to her?		
Emotion	**Emotion**	**Emotion**
What emotion was associated with the automatic thought?		
Behavior	**Behavior**	**Behavior**
What did the patient do then?		

FIGURE 10.1. Cognitive Conceptualization Diagram. Copyright 1993 by Judith S. Beck, Ph.D.

COGNITIVE CONCEPTUALIZATION DIAGRAM

Patient's name: _Sally_ _____ Date: _2/22_ _____

Diagnosis: Axis I _Major depressive episode_   Axis II _None_ _____

Relevant Childhood Data
Compared self with older brother and peers Critical mother

Core Belief(s)
I'm inadequate.

Conditional Assumptions/Beliefs/Rules
(positive) If I work very hard, I can do okay. (negative) If I don't do great, then I've failed.

Compensatory Strategies
Develop high standards   Look for shortcomings and correct Work very hard   Avoid seeking help Overprepare

Situation 1	Situation 2	Situation 3
Talking to freshmen about advanced placement credits	Thinking about course requirements	Reflecting on difficulty of math text

Automatic Thought	Automatic Thought	Automatic Thought
They're all smarter than me.	I won't be able to do it [research paper].	I won't make it through the course.

Meaning of the A.T.	Meaning of the A.T.	Meaning of the A.T.
I'm inadequate.	I'm inadequate.	I'm inadequate.

Emotion	Emotion	Emotion
Sad	Sad	Sad

Behavior	Behavior	Behavior
—	Cried	Closed the book; stopped studying

FIGURE 10.2. Sally's Cognitive Conceptualization Diagram. Copyright 1993 by Judith S. Beck, Ph.D.

To complete the top box of the diagram, the therapist asks himself (and the patient): How did the core belief originate and become maintained? What life events (especially those in childhood) did the patient experience that might be related to the development and maintenance of the belief? Typical relevant childhood data include such significant events as continual or periodic strife among parents or other family members; parental divorce; negative interactions with parents, siblings, teachers, peers, or others in which the child felt blamed, criticized, or otherwise devalued; illness; death of significant others; physical or sexual abuse; and other adverse life conditions, such as growing up in poverty, facing chronic racial discrimination, and so on.

The relevant childhood data may, however, be more subtle: for example, the child's perception (which may or may not have been valid) that parents favored a sibling over her; the child's continual self-criticism over not measuring up in some important way to a sibling; the child's feeling different from or demeaned by peers; or the child's perception that she did not meet expectations of parents, teachers, or others.

Next the therapist asks himself, "How did the patient cope with this painful core belief? What intermediate beliefs (i.e., underlying assumptions, rules, and attitudes) has she developed?"

Sally's beliefs are depicted hierarchically in Figure 10.3. As Sally has many intermediate beliefs that could be classified as attitudes or rules, it is particularly useful to list the key *assumptions* in the box below the core belief. (See p. 149 for how the therapist can help a patient reexpress an attitude or rule as an assumption.) Sally, for example, developed a positive assumption which helped her cope with the painful idea of inadequacy: "If I work very hard, then I can do okay." Like most patients, she also had a negative assumption, which was the flip side of the positive, "If I don't work hard, then I'll fail." Most Axis I patients tend to operate according to their positive assumptions until they become psychologically distressed, at which time the negative assumption surfaces.

To complete the next box, "compensatory strategies," the therapist asks himself, "Which behavioral strategies did the patient develop to cope with the painful core belief?" Note that the patient's broad assumptions often link the compensatory strategies to the core belief: "If I [engage in the compensatory strategy], then [my core belief may not come true]. However, if I [do *not* engage in my compensatory strategy], then [my core belief *may* come true]." Sally's strategies were to develop high standards for herself, work very hard, overprepare for exams and presentations, and be hypervigilant for her shortcomings and avoid seeking help (especially in situations in which asking for assistance could, in her mind, expose her inadequacy). She believes that doing these things will protect her from failure and the exposure of her inadequacy (and

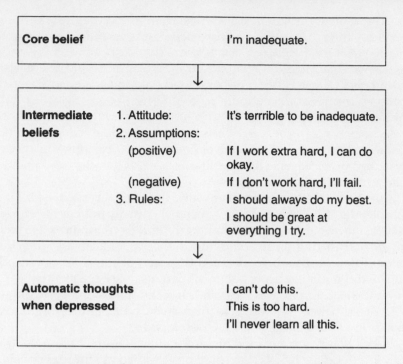

FIGURE 10.3. Hierarchy of beliefs and automatic thoughts.

that not doing these things *could* lead to failure and exposure of inadequacy).

Another patient might have developed strategies that are the opposite of Sally's behaviors: avoiding hard work, developing few goals, underpreparing, and asking for excessive help. Why did Sally develop her set of coping strategies while a second patient developed the opposite set? Perhaps nature endowed them with different cognitive and behavioral styles; in interaction with the environment they developed different intermediate beliefs that reinforced their particular behavioral strategies. The second hypothesized patient, perhaps because of her childhood experiences, had the same core belief of inadequacy but coped with it by developing another set of beliefs: "If I set low goals for myself, I may be able to meet them, and even if I don't meet them, I'll have less to lose"; "If I try minimally and fail, then my failure is due to lack of effort rather than to inadequacy"; "If I rely on myself then I won't be able to accomplish what I need to. Therefore it is better to depend on others." The therapist might explain to this latter patient that her childhood environment in conjunction with her hereditary predisposition may account for the development of her particular beliefs and coping strategies, stressing that through therapy she can learn to override or modify the beliefs and strategies when they prove dysfunctional.

Note that compensatory strategies are *normal* behaviors that everyone engages in at times. The difficulty of patients in distress lies in the *overuse* of these strategies at the expense of more functional strategies. Figure 10.4 lists a few examples of strategies that patients develop to cope with painful core beliefs.

To summarize: The Cognitive Conceptualization Diagram should make logical sense to the therapist and patient. It should be continually reevaluated and refined as additional data are collected. The therapist introduces it to the patient as an explanatory device, designed to help make sense of the patient's current reactions to situations. The therapist may introduce just the bottom half initially, saving the top portion for a time when he judges the patient will benefit. Whereas some patients are intellectually and emotionally ready to see the larger picture early on in therapy, others (especially those who do not have a sound therapeutic relationship or do not really believe in the cognitive model) should be exposed to the diagram much later in therapy (if at all). As mentioned previously, whenever the therapist presents his conceptualization, he asks the patient for confirmation, disconfirmation, or modification of his hypotheses.

Identifying Intermediate Beliefs

How does the therapist identify intermediate beliefs? He does so by:

1. Recognizing when a belief is expressed as an automatic thought.
2. Providing the first part of an assumption.
3. Directly eliciting a rule or attitude.
4. Using the downward arrow technique.
5. Examining the patient's automatic thoughts and looking for common themes.
6. Reviewing a belief questionnaire completed by the patient.

These strategies are illustrated below.

1. First, a patient may actually articulate a belief as an automatic thought, especially if she is depressed:

THERAPIST: What went through your mind when you got the quiz back?

PATIENT: I should have done better. I can't do anything right. I'm so inadequate. [*core belief*]

Avoid negative emotion	Display high emotion (e.g., to attract attention)
Try to be perfect	Purposely appear incompetent or helpless
Be overly responsible	Avoid responsibility
Avoid intimacy	Seek inappropriate intimacy
Seek recognition	Avoid attention
Avoid confrontation	Provoke others
Try to control situations	Abdicate control to others
Act childlike	Act in an authoritarian manner
Try to please others	Distance self from others or try to please only oneself

FIGURE 10.4. Typical compensatory strategies.

2. Second, the therapist may be able to elicit a full assumption by providing the first half of it.

T: So you had the thought, "I'll have to stay up all night working."

P: Yes.

T: And if you don't work as hard as you possibly can on a paper or a project—

P: Then I haven't done my best. I've failed.

T: Does this sound familiar, based on what we've talked about before in therapy? Is this generally how you view your efforts, that if you don't work as hard as you can, then you've failed?

P: Yes, I think so.

T: Can you give me some more examples so we can see how widespread this belief is?

3. Third, the therapist can identify a rule or an attitude by direct elicitation.

T: So it's pretty important to you to do really well in your volunteer tutoring job?

P: Oh, yes.

T: Do you remember our talking about this kind of thing before: having to do very well? Do you have a rule about that?

P: Oh . . . I hadn't really thought of it . . . I guess I have to do whatever I do really well.

4. More often, the therapist uses a fourth technique to identify intermediate (and core) beliefs: the *downward arrow technique* (Burns, 1980). First, the therapist identifies a key automatic thought which he suspects may be directly stemming from a dysfunctional belief. Then he asks the patient for the *meaning* of this cognition, assuming the automatic thought were true. He continues to do so until he has uncovered one or more important beliefs. Asking what a thought means *to* the patient often elicits an intermediate belief; asking what it means *about* the patient usually uncovers the core belief.

T: Okay, to summarize, you were studying late last night, you were looking over your class notes, you had the thought, "These notes stink," and you felt sad.

P: Right.

T: Okay, now we haven't yet looked at the evidence to see if you're right. But I'd like to see if we can figure out *why* that thought made you feel so sad. To do that, we have to assume for a moment that you *are* right, your notes stink. What would that mean to you?

P: I didn't do a very good job in class.

T: Okay, if it's true that you didn't do a very good job in class, what would that mean?

P: I'm a lousy student.

T: Okay, if you're a lousy student, what does that mean about you?

P: I'm not good enough. [I am inadequate.] [*core belief*]

Sometimes the therapist gets stuck in the course of a downward arrow technique when the patient answers with a "feeling" response, such as "That would be terrible," or "I'd be so anxious." As in the example below, the therapist gently empathizes and then tries to get back on track. To minimize the possibility that the patient will react negatively to his probing, the therapist provides a rationale for his repeated questioning and varies his inquiry through questions such as the following:

> "If that's true, so what?"
> "What's so bad about—"
> "What's the worst part about—"
> "What does that mean *about* you?"

The transcript below demonstrates the provision of a brief rationale and the variation of questions in the downward arrow technique.

T: It's important to me to understand the most upsetting part of this to you. What would it mean if your roommates and friends did get better grades than you?

P: Oh, I couldn't stand it.

T: So you'd be pretty upset, but what would be the worst part about it?

P: They'd probably look down on me.

T: And if they did look down on you, what would be so bad about it?

P: I'd hate that.

T: Sure, you'd be distressed if that happened. But so what if they looked down on you?

P: I don't know. That would be pretty bad.

T: Would it mean something *about* you, if they looked down on you?

P: Sure. It'd mean I'm inferior, not as good as they are.

How does the therapist know when to stop the downward arrow technique? Generally the therapist has uncovered the important intermediate beliefs and/or core belief when the patient shows a negative shift in affect and/or begins to state the belief in the same or similar words.

T: And what would it mean if you are inferior and not as good as them?

P: Just that, I'm inferior; I'm inadequate. [*core belief*]

5. A fifth way to identify beliefs is to look for common themes in a patient's automatic thoughts across situations. The therapist can ask an insightful patient whether she can identify a recurrent theme or he can hypothesize a belief and ask the patient to reflect on its validity:

T: Sally, in a number of situations you seem to have the thought, "I can't do it," or "It's too hard," or "I won't be able to get it done." I wonder if you have a belief that you are somehow incompetent or inadequate?

P: Yes, I think I do. I do think I'm inadequate.

6. A sixth way to identify beliefs is to ask the patient directly. Some patients are able to articulate their beliefs fairly easily.

T: Sally, what is your belief about asking for help?

P: Oh, asking for help is a sign of weakness.

7. Finally, a patient may be asked to complete a belief questionnaire such as the Dysfunctional Attitude Scale (Weissman & Beck, 1978). Careful review of items that are very strongly endorsed can highlight problematic beliefs. The use of such questionnaires is a useful adjunct to the techniques described above.

To summarize, the therapist can identify beliefs, both intermediate and core beliefs, in a number of ways:

- Looking for the expression of a belief in an automatic thought.
- Providing the conditional clause ("If . . .) of an assumption and asking the patient to complete it.
- Directly eliciting a rule.
- Using the downward arrow technique.
- Recognizing a common theme among automatic thoughts.
- Asking the patient what she thinks her belief is.
- Reviewing the patient's belief questionnaire.

Deciding Whether to Modify a Belief

Having identified a belief, the therapist determines whether the intermediate belief is central or more peripheral. Generally, in order to conduct therapy as efficiently as possible, he focuses on the most important intermediate beliefs (Safran, Vallis, Segal, & Shaw, 1986). The therapist's time and effort can be wasted by working on dysfunctional beliefs that are tangential or by working on a belief that the patient believes only slightly.

T: It sounds as if you believe if people don't accept you, then you're inferior.

P: I guess.

T: How much do you believe that?

P: Not that much, maybe 20%.

T: It doesn't sound as if we have to work on that belief, then. How about if we get back to the problem we were discussing before?

Having identified an important intermediate belief, the therapist decides whether he will make the belief explicit to the patient and, if so, whether he will merely identify the belief as one to be worked on in the future or whether they will work on it at the present time. To help him decide among these options, the therapist asks himself:

- What is the belief?
- How strongly does the patient believe it?
- If strongly, how broadly does it affect her life? How strongly does it affect her life?
- If strongly, should I work on it now? Is the patient ready to work on it? Is it likely she will be able to evaluate it with sufficient objectivity at this point? Do we have enough time in the session today to begin work on it? Does it fit into the items left on our agenda or will the patient be amenable to postponing discussion of our agenda item to make time for us to explore this belief?

Generally the therapist refrains from belief modification until the patient has learned the tools to identify and modify her automatic thoughts and has gained some symptom relief. Belief modification is relatively easy with some patients and much more difficult with others. Modification of intermediate beliefs is generally accomplished before modification of core beliefs as the latter may be quite rigid.

Educating Patients about Beliefs

Having identified an important belief and having checked that the patient believes it strongly, the therapist may decide to educate the patient about the nature of beliefs in general, using a specific belief as an example. He stresses that there are a range of potential beliefs that the patient could adopt and that beliefs are learned, not innate, and so can be revised.

T: Okay, so we've identified some of your beliefs: "It's terrible to do a mediocre job." "I have to do everything great." "If I do less than my best, I'm a failure." Where do you think you learned these ideas?

P: Growing up, I guess.

T: Does everyone have these same beliefs?

P: No. Some people don't seem to care.

T: Can you think of someone specifically who seems to have different beliefs?

P: Well, my cousin Emily, for one.

T: What belief does she have?

P: I think she thinks it's okay to be mediocre. She's more interested in having a good time.

T: So she learned different beliefs?

P: I guess so.

T: Well, the bad news is that you currently have a set of beliefs which aren't bringing you much satisfaction, right? The good news is that since you *learned* this current set of beliefs, you can unlearn them and learn others—maybe not as extreme as Emily's, but somewhere in between hers and yours. How does that sound?

P: Good.

Changing Rules and Attitudes into Assumption Form

It is often easier for patients to see the distortion in and test an intermediate belief that is in the form of an assumption rather than a rule or an attitude. Having identified a rule or an attitude, the therapist uses the downward arrow technique to ascertain its meaning.

T: So you believe pretty strongly that you should do things yourself [*rule*] and that it's terrible to ask for help [*attitude*]. What does it mean to you to ask for help, for example with your schoolwork, instead of doing it yourself?

P: It means I'm inadequate.

T: How much do you believe this idea right now, "If I ask for help, I'm inadequate?"

Logical evaluation of this conditional assumption through questioning or other methods often creates greater cognitive dissonance than does evaluation of the rule or attitude. It is easier for Sally to recognize the distortion and/or dysfunctionality in the assumption, "If I ask for help, it means I'm incompetent," than in her rule, "I shouldn't ask for help."

Examining Advantages and Disadvantages of Beliefs

Often it is useful for patients to examine the advantages and disadvantages of continuing to hold a given belief. The therapist then strives to minimize or undermine the advantages and emphasize and reinforce the disadvantages. (A similar process was previously described in the section on evaluating the utility of automatic thoughts in Chapter 8, pp. 120–121.)

T: What are the *advantages* of believing if you don't do your best then you're a failure?

P: Well, it might make me work harder.

T: It'd be interesting to see if you actually *need* such an extreme belief to keep you working hard. We'll get back to that idea later. Any other advantages?

P: . . . No, not that I can think of.

T: What are the *disadvantages* of believing you're a failure if you don't do your best?

P: Well, I feel miserable when I don't do well on an exam. . . . I get really nervous before presentations. . . . I don't have as much time to do other things I like because I'm so busy studying—

T: And does it cut some enjoyment out of studying and learning itself?

P: Oh, definitely.

T: Okay, so on one hand, it may or may not actually be true that this belief is the only thing that makes you work hard. On the other hand, this belief about having to live up to your potential makes you feel miserable when you don't do great, makes you more nervous than you have to be before presentations, cuts into your enjoyment of your work and stops you from doing other things you like. Is that right?

P: Yes.

T: Is this an idea, then, that you'd like to change?

Formulating a New Belief

In order to decide which strategies to use to modify a given belief, the therapist clearly formulates to himself a more adaptive belief. He asks himself, "What belief would be more functional for the patient?"

For example, Figure 10.5 lists Sally's current beliefs and the new beliefs the therapist has in mind. Although constructing a new belief is a *collaborative* process, the therapist nevertheless mentally formulates a range of more reasonable beliefs so he can appropriately choose strategies to change the old belief.

To summarize, before the therapist tries to modify a patient's belief, he confirms that it is a central, strongly held belief and he formulates in his own mind a more functional, less rigid belief that is thematically *related* to the dysfunctional one, but which he believes would result in greater satisfaction for the patient. He does not impose this belief on the patient but rather guides the patient in a collaborative manner, using Socratic questioning, to construct an alternative belief. He may, in addition, educate the patient about the nature of beliefs (e.g., that they are ideas, not necessarily truths; that they have been learned and so can be unlearned; that they can be evaluated and modified) and/or help the patient assess the advantages and disadvantages of continuing to hold the belief.

Sally's old beliefs	More functional beliefs
1. If I don't do as well as others, I'm a failure.	If I don't do as well as others, I'm not a failure, just human.
2. If I ask for help, it's a sign of weakness.	If I ask for help when I need it, I'm showing good problem-solving abilities (which is a sign of strength).
3. If I fail at work/school, I'm a failure as a person.	If I fail at work/school, it's not a reflection of my whole self. (My whole self includes how I am as a friend, daughter, sister, relative, citizen, and community member, and my qualities of kindness, sensitivity to others, helpfulness, etc.) Also, failure is not a permanent condition.
4. I should be able to excel at everything I try.	I shouldn't be able to excel at something unless I am gifted in that area (and am willing and able to devote considerable time and effort to it at the expense of other things).
5. I should always work hard and do my best.	I should put in a reasonable amount of effort much of the time.
6. If I don't live up to my potential, I have failed.	If I do less than my best, I have succeeded perhaps 70%, 80%, or 90%; not 0%.
7. If I don't work hard all the time, I'll fail.	If I don't work hard all the time I'll probably do reasonably well and have a more balanced life.

FIGURE 10.5. Formulation of more functional beliefs.

MODIFYING BELIEFS

Listed below are common strategies for modifying both intermediate and core beliefs. (Additional techniques for modifying core beliefs are presented in more detail in the next chapter.) Some beliefs may change easily but many take concerted effort over a period of time. The therapist continues to ask the patient how much she currently believes a given belief (0–100%) in order to gauge whether further work is needed.

It is usually neither possible nor necessarily desirable to reduce the degree of belief to 0%. Knowing when to stop working on a belief is therefore a judgment call. Generally, a belief has been sufficiently attenuated when the patient endorses it less than 30% and when she is likely to continue to modify her dysfunctional behavior despite still holding onto a remnant of the belief.

It is advisable for patients to keep track of the beliefs they have explored in their therapy notes. A useful format includes the dysfunctional belief, the new, more functional belief, and the strength of each belief, expressed in a percentage, as in the following example:

> *Old belief:* If I don't achieve highly, I'm a failure. (55%)
> *New belief:* I'm only an overall failure if I acutally fail at almost everything. (80%)

A typical homework assignment is to read and rerate daily how strongly the patient endorses both beliefs each day.

Some of the strategies used to modify beliefs are the same as those used to modify automatic thoughts, but there are additional techniques as well, including:

> 1. Socratic questioning
> 2. Behavioral experiments
> 3. Cognitive continuum
> 4. Rational–emotional role-plays
> 5. Using others as a reference point
> 6. Acting "as if"
> 7. Self-disclosure

Socratic Questioning to Modify Beliefs

As illustrated in the next transcript, the therapist uses the same kinds of questions to examine Sally's belief that he used in evaluating her automatic thoughts. Even when he identifies a general belief, he helps her evaluate it in the context of specific situations. This specifity helps make the evaluation more concrete and meaningful, and less abstract and intellectual.

T: (*Summarizing what they learned from the just completed downward arrow technique.*) Okay, so you believe about 90% that if you ask for help, it means you're inadequate. Is that right?

P: Yes.

T: Could there be another way of viewing asking for help?

P: I'm not sure.

T: Take therapy, for example. Are you inadequate because you came for help here?

P: A little, maybe.

T: Hmmm. That's interesting to me because I usually view it in the opposite way. Is it possible it's actually a sign of strength and adequacy that you came to therapy? Because what would have happened if you hadn't?

P: I might still be pulling the covers over my head, not going to class.

T: Are you suggesting that asking for appropriate help when you have an illness like depression is a more adequate thing to do than remaining depressed?

P: Yeah . . . I guess so.

T: Well, you tell me. Let's say we have two depressed college students. One seeks treatment and the other doesn't but continues to have depressive symptoms. Which do you consider more adequate?

P: Well, the one who goes for help.

T: Now how about another situation you've mentioned—your volunteer job. Again, we have two college students, this is their first tutoring experience; they are unsure of what to do because they've never done it before. One seeks help, the other doesn't, but continues to struggle. Who's the more adequate?

P: (*Hesitantly.*) The one who goes for help?

T: Are you sure?

P: (*Thinks for a moment.*) Yeah. It's not a sign of adequacy to just struggle if you could get help and do better.

T: How much do you believe that?

P: Pretty much: 80%.

T: And how do these two situations—therapy and help in tutoring—apply to you?

P: I guess they do.

T: Let's have you write something down about this. . . . Let's call the first idea "old belief"—now what did you say?

P: If I ask for help, I'm inadequate.

T: And let's see, you believed it 90% before. Put "90%" next to it. And how much do you believe it now? . . . The same amount? More? Less?

P: Less. Maybe 40%.

T: Okay, write "40%" next to the "90%."

P: (*Does so.*)

T: Now, write "new belief." How would you put that?

P: If I ask for help, I'm not inadequate?

T: You could put that. Or how about, "If I ask for help when it's reasonable, it's a sign of adequacy."

P: Okay. (*Writes that.*)

T: How much do you believe the new belief now?

P: A lot. . . . (*Reads and ponders the new belief.*) Maybe 70 to 80%. (*Writes that down.*)

T: Okay, Sally, we'll be coming back to these beliefs again. How about for homework this week if you do two things? One is to read these beliefs every day and rate how much you believe them—actually write down the percentage next to the beliefs themselves.

P: Okay.

T: Writing down how much you believe them will make you really think about them. That's why I didn't say just read them.

P: Okay. (*Writes down the assignment.*)

T: Second, could you be on the lookout for other situations this week where you *could* reasonably ask for help? That is, let's imagine that you believe the new belief 100%, that asking for reasonable help *is* a sign of adequacy. When during this coming week might you ask for help? Jot down those situations.

P: Okay.

In the previous segment, the therapist uses Socratic questioning in the context of specific situations to help Sally evaluate an intermediate belief. He judges that the standard questions of examining the evidence and evaluating outcomes will be less effective than leading Sally to develop an alternative viewpoint. His questions are much more persuasive and less evenhanded than when he helps her evaluate more malleable cognitions at the automatic thought level. A follow-up homework assignment is designed to have her continue to reflect daily on both the dysfunctional assumption and the new belief.

Behavioral Experiments to Test Beliefs

As with automatic thoughts, the therapist can help the patient devise a behavioral test to evaluate the validity of a belief (see also Chapter 12, pp. 197–200). Behavioral experiments, properly designed and carried out, can modify a patient's beliefs more powerfully than verbal techniques in the office.

T: Okay, Sally, we've identified another belief: "If I ask for help, others will belittle me," and you believe that 60%. Of course, I haven't actually belittled you, have I?

P: No, of course not. But that's your job, to help people.

T: True, but it would be useful to find out if other people, in general, are more like me or not. How could you find out?

P: Ask other people for help, I guess.

T: Okay, whom could you ask and for what kind of help?

P: Ummm. I'm not sure.

T: How about if we make a list of some of the possibilities? I'll go first; maybe that'll help jog some of your ideas. After we have a list, you can decide whom you'd like to test this idea with.

P: Okay.

T: Could you ask your roommate?

P: Yeah, actually I already do. And I could ask my resident adviser for help with something.

T: Good. How about your academic adviser?

P: Uh huh. I could also ask my brother. No. I won't ask my roommate or my brother. I know they wouldn't belittle me.

T: Oh, so you know already there are some exceptions?

P: Yes. But I guess I could go to my adviser or my teaching assistants.

T: What could you ask for help with?

P: Well, the teaching assistants . . . I could ask questions about the papers I have due or about the readings. The resident adviser, I don't know. My academic adviser . . . I would feel a little funny going to her. I don't really even know what I want to major in.

T: That would be an interesting experiment—going for help in deciding a major to the person whose job it is to help students make those kinds of decisions.

P: True—

T: So you might kill two birds with one stone—testing the belief that you'll be belittled *and* getting some guidance for a real-life problem you have.

P: I guess I could.

T: Good. So would you like to test the belief, "If I ask others for help, they'll belittle me?" How would you like to do that this week?

In the previous segment, the therapist suggests a behavioral experiment to test a belief. Had he sensed hesitation on the patient's part, he would probably ask her how likely she was to do the experiment and what practical problems or thoughts might get in her way. He might also have her do covert rehearsal (see Chapter 14, pp. 257–259) to increase the likelihood of her following through. In addition, if he judged that there was the possibility of others' belittling Sally, he might have discussed in advance what such belittling would mean to her and how she could cope if the belittling did occur. Also, he might have asked Sally for a description of belittling to ensure that she would not inaccurately perceive others' behavior as belittling when they did not intend it to be.

Cognitive Continuum to Modify Beliefs

This technique is useful to modify both automatic thoughts and beliefs that reflect polarized thinking (i.e., when the patient sees something in all-or-nothing terms). Sally, for example, believed that if she was not a superior student, she was a failure. Building a cognitive continuum for the concept in question facilitates the patient's recognition of the middle ground, as the following transcript illustrates:

T: Okay, you believe pretty strongly that if you're not a superior student, you're a failure. Let's see what that looks like graphically. (*Draws a number line.*)

	Initial Graph of Success	
0% Success	90%	100% Success
Sally		Superior student

T: Now, where does the superior student go?

P: Up here. I guess 90–100%.

T: Okay. And, you're a failure. Are you at 0% success then?

P: I guess.

T: Are you also saying everything from 90% down equals a failure?

P: Maybe not.

T: Okay, where does failure start?

P: Around 50%, I guess.

T: 50%? Then, everyone who falls below 50% is a failure?

P: I'm not sure.

T: Now, is there anyone else who more realistically belongs at 0% than you?

P: Ummm . . . Maybe this guy, Jack, who's in my economics class. I know he's doing worse than I am.

T: Okay. We'll put Jack at 0%. But, I wonder if there is anyone who's doing even worse than Jack?

P: Probably.

T: Is it conceivable that there is someone who is failing every test, every paper?

P: Yeah.

T: Okay, now if we put that person at 0%, a real failure, where does that put Jack? Where does that put you?

P: Probably Jack's at 30%. And I'm at 50%.

T: Now, how about a person who is failing everything but he isn't even showing up at any classes or doing any of the reading or turning in any papers?

P: I guess *he* would be at 0%.

T: Where does that put the student who is at least trying but not passing?

P: I guess he would be at 10%.

T: Where does that put you and Jack?

P: Jack goes to about 50%; I guess I'm at 75%.

Revised Success–Failure Graph					
0%	10%	50%	75%	90%	100%
Student who does nothing	Student who tries but gets failing grades	Jack	Sally	Superior students	

T: How about for homework if you see whether even 75% is accurate? Even if it is for this school, perhaps for schools and students in general, you would rank higher. In any case, how accurate is it to call someone a failure who is at the 75% mark?

P: Not very.

T: Maybe the *worst* thing you can say is that she is 75% successful.

P: Yeah. (*Brightens visibly.*)

T: Okay, to get back to your original idea, how much do you believe now that if you are not a superior student, you are a failure?

P: Not as much. Maybe 25%.

T: Good!

The cognitive continuum technique is often useful when the patient is displaying dichotomous thinking. As with most techniques, the therapist may directly teach the patient how to employ the technique herself so she can use it when it is applicable.

T: Sally, let's review what we did here. We identified an all-or-nothing error in your thinking. Then we drew a number line to see whether there were really only two categories—success and failure—or whether it's more accurate to consider *degrees* of success. Can you think of anything else that you see in only two categories and that distresses you?

Rational–Emotional Role-Play

This technique, also called point–counterpoint (Young, 1990), is usually employed after the therapist has tried other techniques such as those described in this chapter. It is particularly useful when a patient says that *intellectually* she can see that a belief is dysfunctional but that *emotionally* or in her gut it still "feels" true. The therapist first provides a rationale for asking the patient to play the "emotional" part of her mind that strongly endorses the dysfunctional belief, while he, the therapist, plays the "rational" part. In the second segment they switch roles. Note in both segments patient and therapist speak as the patient; that is, they both use the word "I."

T: It sounds from what you're saying that you still believe to some extent that you're inadequate because you didn't do as well in school last semester as you would have liked.

P: Yeah.

T: I'd like to get a better sense of what evidence you still have that supports your belief.

P: Okay.

T: What I'd like to do is a role-play. I'll play the "rational" part of your mind which intellectually knows that just because you didn't get all A's doesn't mean you are inadequate through and through. I'd like you to play the "emotional" part of your mind, that voice from your gut that still really believes you *are* inadequate. I want you to argue against me as hard as you can so I can really see what's maintaining the belief. Okay?

P: Yeah.

T: Okay, you start. Say "I'm inadequate because I didn't get all A's."

P: I'm inadequate because I didn't get all A's.

T: No, I'm not. I have a *belief* that I'm inadequate, but I am reasonably adequate most of the time.

P: No, I'm not. If I were truly adequate, I *would* have gotten all A's last semester.

T: That's not true. Adequacy doesn't equal total academic perfection. If that were true, only 1% of the students in the world would be adequate and everyone else would be inadequate.

P: Well, I got a C in chemistry. That *proves* I'm inadequate.

T: That's not right either. If I had flunked the course *perhaps* it might be reasonable to say I wasn't adequate in chemistry, but it doesn't make me inadequate in *everything*. Besides, maybe I really am adequate in chemistry, but I flunked for other reasons; for example, I was depressed and couldn't concentrate on my studying.

P: But a truly adequate person wouldn't become depressed in the first place.

T: Actually, even truly adequate people get depressed. There isn't a connection there. And when truly adequate people get depressed, their concentration and motivation definitely suffer, and they don't perform as well as usual. But that doesn't mean they are inadequate through and through.

P: I guess that's true. They're just depressed.

T: You're right, but you're out of role. Any more evidence that you're completely inadequate?

P: (*Thinks for a moment.*) No, I guess not.

T: Well, how about if we trade roles now and this time you be the "rational" part who disputes my "emotional" part? And I'll use your same arguments.

P: Okay.

T: I'll start. "I'm inadequate because I don't get all A's."

Switching roles provides the patient with an opportunity to voice the rational arguments just modeled by the therapist. The therapist uses the same emotional reasoning that the patient used and tries to use the same words, as well. Using the patient's own words and not introducing new material helps the patient to respond more precisely to her specific concerns.

If the patient is unable to formulate a response while in the rational role, patient and therapist can either switch roles temporarily or they can both come out of role to discuss the stuck point. As with any belief modification technique, the therapist evaluates both its effectiveness and the degree to which the patient needs further work on the belief. He does so by asking the patient to rate how much she believes the belief after the intervention.

Many patients find the rational–emotional role-play useful. A few, however, feel uncomfortable doing it. As with any intervention, the decision to use it should be collaborative. Because it is a more argumentative technique than most, the therapist takes care to avoid the patient's perceiving it as confrontational by watching for her nonverbal reactions during the role-play. He also takes care to make sure that the patient does not feel criticized or denigrated by his elevation of the rational part of her mind over the emotional part.

Using Other People as a Reference Point in Belief Modification

When patients consider *other* people's beliefs, they often get psychological distance from their own dysfunctional beliefs. They begin to see an inconsistency between what they believe is true or right for themselves and what they more objectively believe is true about other people. Following are four examples of using other people as a reference point to gain distance.

Example 1

T: Sally, you mentioned last week that you think your cousin Emily has a different belief about having to do everything great.

P: Yeah.

T: Could you put what you think her belief is into words?

P: She thinks she doesn't have to do great. She's an okay person, no matter what.

T: Do you believe she's right? That she doesn't have to do great to be an okay person?

P: Oh, yes.

T: Do you see her as inadequate, through and through?

P: Oh, no. She might not get good grades but she's certainly adequate.

T: I wonder if Emily's belief could apply to you: "If I don't do great, I'm still an okay, adequate person."

P: Hmmm.

T: Is there something different about Emily that makes her okay and adequate no matter how well or poorly she does, but not you?

P: (*Thinks for a moment.*) No. I don't think so. I guess I hadn't really thought of it that way.

T: How much do you believe right now, "If I don't do great, I'm inadequate"?

P: Less, maybe 60%.

T: And how much do you believe this new belief, "If I don't do great, I'm still an okay, adequate person"?

P: More than before. Maybe 70%.

T: Good. How about if we have you write down the new belief, and start making a list of the evidence that supports this new belief.

At this point, the therapist might introduce the Core Belief Worksheet, described in Chapter 11, which can be used for both core beliefs and intermediate beliefs.

Example 2

Another way to help the patient modify an intermediate or core belief is to have her identify someone else who plainly seems to have the same dysfunctional belief. Sometimes the patient can see the distortion in someone else's belief and apply this insight to herself. This technique is analogous to the Dysfunctional Thought Record question: "If [friend's name] was in this situation and had this thought, what would I tell [him/her]?"

T: Do you know anyone else who you think has your same belief, "If I don't work hard, I'll fail"?

P: I'm sure my friend, Donna, from high school, believes that. She's always studying, night and day.

T: How accurate do you think that belief is for her?

P: Oh, not at all. She's very bright. She probably couldn't fail if she tried.

T: Is it possible that she might consider anything less than an A a failure, too?

P: Yes, I know she does.

T: And do you agree with her, that if she gets a B, then she's failed?

P: No, of course not.

T: How would you view it?

P: She got a B. An okay grade, not the best, but not a *failure*.

T: What belief would you like her to have?

P: It's good to work hard and try for A's but it's not the end of the world if you don't get them. And it doesn't mean you've failed.

T: How does all this apply to you?

P: Hmmm. I guess it's the same.

T: Could you spell out what's the same?

P: That if I don't get all A's, I haven't failed. I still think I should work hard, though.

T: Sure. It's reasonable to want to work hard and do well. The unreasonable part is to believe you've failed if you haven't done perfectly. Do you agree with that?

Example 3

The therapist could also do a role-play with the patient in which he instructs her to convince another person that the belief they both share is invalid for the other person.

T: Sally, you say you think your roommate also believes that she shouldn't go to a professor for help because he might think she's unprepared or not smart enough?

P: Yes.

T: Do you agree with her?

P: No. She's probably wrong. But even if he is critical, it doesn't mean he's right.

T: Could we try to role-play this? I'll be your roommate; you give me advice. Don't let me get away with any distorted thinking.

P: Okay.

T: I'll start. Sally, I don't understand this stuff. What should I do?

P: Go to the professor.

T: Oh, I couldn't do that. He'll think I'm dumb. He'll think I'm wasting his time.

P: Hey, it's his job to help students.

T: But he probably doesn't like students bothering him.

P: Tough, that's what he's getting paid for. Anyway, good professors like to help students. If he's impatient, that says something about him, not about you.

T: But even if he doesn't mind helping, he'll find out how confused I am.

P: That's okay. He won't expect you to know everything. That's why you're coming to him.

T: What if he thinks I'm dumb?

P: First of all, you wouldn't be here if you were dumb. Second, if he does expect you to know everything, he's just wrong. If you did know everything, you wouldn't be taking his course.

T: I still think I shouldn't go.

P: No, you should. Don't let his snobby attitude make you feel like you're imposing or you're dumb. You're not.

T: Okay. I'm convinced. Out of role, how does what you told your roommate apply to you?

Example 4

Finally, many patients can get distance from a belief by using their own children as a reference point or by imagining that they have children.

T: Sally, so you believe 80% that if you don't do as well as everyone else then you've failed?

P: Yeah.

T: I wonder, can you imagine that you have a daughter? She's 10 years old and in fifth grade, and she comes home one day very, very upset because her friends got A's on a test and she got a C. Would you want her to believe that she's a failure?

P: No, of course not.

T: Why not? . . . What would you like her to believe? (*The patient responds.*) Now how does what you've just said apply to you?

Acting "As If"

Changes in belief often lead to corresponding changes in behavior. And changes in behavior, in turn, often lead to corresponding changes in belief. If a belief is fairly weak, the patient may be able to change a target behavior easily and quickly, without much cognitive intervention. Many beliefs do require some modification before the patient is willing to change behaviorally. However, frequently only *some* belief modification, not complete belief change, is needed. And once the patient begins to change her behavior, the belief itself becomes somewhat more attenuated (which makes it easier to continue the new behavior, which further attenuates the belief, and so on, in a positive upward spiral).

T: Okay, Sally, how much do you believe *now* that it's a sign of weakness to ask for help?

P: Not as much. Maybe 50%.

T: That's a good drop. Would it be to your benefit to act as if you don't believe it at all?

P: I'm not sure what you mean.

T: If you didn't believe it was a sign of weakness, in fact, if you believed it was *good* to ask for help, what might you do this week?

P: Well, we've been talking about my going to see the teaching assistant. I guess if I really believed it was *good* to ask for help, I would go.

T: Anything else?

P: Well, I might try to find a tutor for economics. . . . I might ask to borrow notes from the guy down the hall—

T: Hey, that's good. And what positive things could happen if you did some of these things?

P: (*Laughs.*) I could get the help that I need.

T: Do you think you're ready this week to act as if you believe it's a good thing to ask for help?

P: Maybe.

T: Okay, in a minute, we'll find out what thoughts might get in the way, but first, how about if you jot down those ideas you had. And do you want to write down this technique to get you going? Act *as if* you believe the new belief, even if you don't totally.

This acting "as if" technique is equally applicable to core beliefs as were the preceding intermediate belief modification techniques.

Using Self-Disclosure to Modify Beliefs

Appropriate and judicious self-disclosure by the therapist can help some patients view their problems or beliefs in a different way. The self-disclosure, of course, should be genuine and relevant.

T: You know, Sally, when I was in college, I had some trouble going to professors for help because I thought I'd be showing my ignorance, too. And to tell you the truth, the few times I did end up doing it anyway, I had mixed results. Sometimes the professors were really nice and helpful. But a couple of times, they were pretty brusque, just told me to reread a chapter or something. The point is, just because I didn't understand something didn't mean I was inadequate. And the professors who were brusque—well, I think that said a lot more about them than about me. What do you think?

In summary, the therapist helps the patient to *identify* intermediate beliefs by recognizing when a belief has been expressed as an automatic thought, by providing part of an assumption, by directly eliciting a rule or an attitude, by using the downward arrow technique, by looking for common themes among the patient's automatic thoughts, and/or by reviewing a belief questionnaire completed by the patient. The therapist next determines how *important* the belief is by ascertaining how strongly the patient believes it and how broadly and strongly it affects her functioning. Then he decides whether to begin the task of *modifying* it in the current session or to wait for future sessions. When beginning belief modification work, the therapist *educates* the patient about the nature of beliefs, *changes rules and attitudes into assumption form,* and explores the *advantages and disadvantages* of a given belief. He mentally *formulates a new, more functional belief* and guides the patient toward its adoption through many *belief modification techniques,* including Socratic questioning, behavioral experiments, cognitive continua, rational–emotional role-plays, using others as a reference point, acting "as if," and self-disclosure. These techniques are often somewhat more persuasive than standard Socratic questioning of automatic thoughts because the beliefs are much more rigidly held. These same techniques can also be used to modify core beliefs.

Chapter 11

CORE BELIEFS

Core beliefs, as described in Chapter 2, are one's most central ideas about the self. Some authors refer to these beliefs as schemas. Beck (1964) differentiates the two by suggesting that schemas are cognitive structures within the mind, the specific content of which are core beliefs. Further, he theorizes that negative core beliefs essentially fall into two broad categories: those associated with helplessness and those associated with unlovability (Beck, in press). Some patients have core beliefs that fall in one category; others have core beliefs in both categories.

These beliefs develop in childhood as the child interacts with significant others and encounters a series of situations. For most of their lives, most people may maintain relatively positive core beliefs (e.g., "I am substantially in control"; "I can do most things competently"; "I am a functional human being"; "I am likable"; "I am worthwhile"). Negative core beliefs may surface only during times of psychological distress. (Some personality disorder patients, however, may have almost continuously activated negative core beliefs.) Often, unlike automatic thoughts, the core belief that patients "know" to be true about themselves is not fully articulated until the therapist peels back the layers by continuing to ask for the meaning of the patient's thoughts as in the downward arrow exercise mentioned earlier.

It is important to note that patients may also have negative core beliefs about other people and their worlds: "Other people are untrustworthy"; "Other people will hurt me"; "The world is a rotten place." Fixed, overgeneralized ideas such as these often need to be evaluated and modified in addition to core beliefs about the self.

Sally, as described earlier, did see herself as competent and likable most of the time. It was not until she became depressed that a latent belief, "I'm inadequate," became activated. Her therapist determined that they should work directly on modifying this core belief, not only to alleviate her current depression but also to prevent or reduce the severity of future episodes.

Negative core beliefs are usually global, overgeneralized, and absolute. When a core belief is activated, the patient is easily able to process information that supports it, but she often fails to recognize or distorts information that is contrary to it. Sally, for example, basically saw herself in a realistically positive, balanced way until she became depressed. Then she believed almost completely that she was inadequate. Any evidence to the contrary, such as her competent performance in some of her classes, was ignored or discounted: "Doing well in English lit doesn't mean I'm adequate; it just comes easily to me." Evidence supporting her belief about inadequacy, however, was readily processed and then overgeneralized: "Getting a C on my economics quiz shows how inadequate I am."

As emphasized throughout this volume, the therapist begins to formulate a conceptualization (including core beliefs) from the beginning of therapy. He does so mentally at first or privately on paper. At some point in therapy he shares his conceptualization with the patient, presenting it as a hypothesis and asking if it "rings true" to her.

In order to decide when and how much of his conceptualization to share with a patient, the therapist considers the following: how strong their therapeutic alliance is, how strongly the patient believes the cognitive model, how activated her core beliefs are in session, how much insight she already has, how concrete her thinking is, and so forth. So, although the therapist has been conceptualizing the patient's core beliefs from the beginning, he carefully chooses when and how he will share his understanding with the patient. Likewise, he chooses when and how he will try to start modifying the core belief. Therapists generally teach patients to learn the tools of identifying, evaluating, and adaptively responding to automatic thoughts and intermediate beliefs before using the same tools for core beliefs.

At times, however, the therapist and patient unwittingly try to evaluate a core belief early in therapy because it has been expressed as an automatic thought. Such evaluation often has little effect. In another case, the therapist may intentionally test the modifiability of a core belief even before they have done much work at the automatic thought and intermediate belief level.

The degree of difficulty in identifying and modifying core beliefs varies from patient to patient. In general, patients who are in significant emotional distress are more easily able than others to express their core beliefs (because the beliefs are activated in session). And, in general, it is far easier to modify the negative core beliefs of Axis I patients whose counterbalancing positive core beliefs have been activated throughout much of their lives. Negative core beliefs of personality disorder patients are usually much more difficult to modify (Beck et al., 1990; Young, 1990) because they typically have fewer positive core beliefs and they have developed a multitude of negative core beliefs that interconnect, supporting each other like a network.

In identifying and modifying core beliefs, the therapist does the following during the course of therapy (each step is described later in this chapter):

1. Mentally hypothesizes from which category of core belief ("helplessness" or "unlovability") specific automatic thoughts appear to have arisen.

2. Specifies the core belief (to himself) using the same techniques he uses to identify the patient's intermediate beliefs.

3. Presents his hypothesis about the core belief(s) to the patient, asking for confirmation or disconfirmation; refines his hypothesis about the core belief as the patient provides additional data about current and childhood situations and her reactions to them.

4. Educates the patient about core beliefs in general and about her specific core belief; guides the patient in monitoring the operation of the core belief in the present.

5. Begins to evaluate and modify the core belief with the patient; assists the patient in specifying a new, more adaptive core belief; examines the childhood origin of the core belief, its maintenance through the years, and its contribution to the patient's present difficulties; continues to monitor the activation of the core belief in the present; uses "rational" methods to decrease the strength of the old core belief and to increase the strength of the new core belief; and uses experiential or "emotional" techniques with heightened affect when the patient no longer strongly believes a core belief "rationally" or "intellectually" but still believes it "emotionally."

CATEGORIZING CORE BELIEFS

As mentioned previously, patients' core beliefs may be categorized in the helplessness realm, the unlovability realm, or both. Whenever the patient presents data (problems, automatic thoughts, emotions, behavior, history), the therapist "listens" for the category of core belief that seems to have been activated. For example, when Sally expresses thoughts about her work being too hard, about her inability to concentrate, and about her fears of failing, her therapist hypothesizes that a core belief in the helpless category was operating. (Another patient consistently expresses thoughts of others not caring about her and fears that she is too different from others to sustain a future relationship. This patient has a core belief in the category of unlovability.)

The top of Figure 11.1 lists typical core beliefs in the helpless category. Themes include being personally helpless (powerless, vulnerable, trapped, out of control, weak, needy) and not measuring up in terms of achievement (failure, inferior, not good enough, loser, disrespected).

The bottom of Figure 11.1 lists typical core beliefs in the unlovable category. Themes include being unworthy, undesirable, and not measuring up (not in achievement but rather in being defective in some way so as to preclude gaining the sustained love and caring of others).

Sometimes it is clear in which category a given core belief belongs, especially when the patient actually uses words such as "I am helpless," or "I am unlovable." At other times, the therapist may not know initially which category of core belief has been activated. For example, a depressed patient says, "I'm not good enough." The therapist then needs

---

Helpless core beliefs

I am helpless.	I am inadequate.
I am powerless.	I am ineffective.
I am out of control.	I am incompetent.
I am weak.	I am a failure.
I am vulnerable.	I am disrespected.
I am needy.	I am defective (i.e., I do not measure up to others).
I am trapped.	I am not good enough (in terms of achievement).

Unlovable core beliefs

I am unlovable.	I am unworthy.
I am unlikable.	I am different.
I am undesirable.	I am defective (i.e., so others will not love me).
I am unattractive.	I am not good enough (to be loved by others).
I am unwanted.	I am bound to be rejected.
I am uncared for.	I am bound to be abandoned.
I am bad.	I am bound to be alone.

FIGURE 11.1. Categories of core beliefs. Copyright 1995 by Judith S. Beck, Ph.D.

to ascertain the meaning of the thought to determine whether the patient believes she is not good enough to achieve or to gain respect (helpless category) or if she is not good enough for others to love her (unlovable category).

To summarize, the therapist begins mentally to formulate a hypothesis about a patient's core beliefs whenever the patient provides data in the form of her reactions to situations (automatic thoughts and their associated meanings, emotions, and behaviors). He first makes a gross distinction (to himself) between cognitions that seem to fall in the helpless category and those in the unlovable category.

IDENTIFYING CORE BELIEFS

The therapist uses the same techniques to identify the patient's specific core belief that he used to identify her intermediate beliefs (see Chapter 10). In addition to the *downward arrow* technique, he looks for *central themes in the patient's automatic thoughts*, watches for *core beliefs expressed as automatic thoughts*, and *directly elicits* the core belief.

The therapist often identifies a core belief early in therapy in order to conceptualize the patient and plan therapy. He may gather data about and even try to help the patient evaluate the core belief early in therapy. In many cases, such early evaluation is ineffective but helps the therapist test the strength, breadth, and modifiability of the core belief.

THERAPIST: What went through your mind when you couldn't finish the statistics assignment?

PATIENT: I can't do anything right. I'll never be able to make it here.

T: And if that's true, that you can't do anything right and you can't make it here, what does that mean? [*downward arrow technique*]

P: I'm hopeless. I'm so inadequate. [*core belief*]

T: How much do you believe you're inadequate?

P: Oh, 100%.

T: And how inadequate are you, a little, a lot?

P: Completely. I'm completely inadequate.

T: In every way?

P: Just about.

T: Any evidence that you're not inadequate?

P: No. . . . No, I don't think so.

T: Did you say you're doing okay in your other courses?

P: Yeah, but not as well as I should be.

T: Does the fact that you're doing okay in them contradict this idea that you're inadequate?

P: No, if I were really adequate, I'd be doing much better.

T: How about other areas of your life—managing your apartment, managing your finances, taking care of yourself . . . ?

P: I'm doing pretty badly at them, too.

T: So this idea that you're inadequate extends to other things, too?

P: Just about everything.

T: Okay, I can see how strongly you believe this idea now. We'll come back to it another time.

Here the therapist uses the downward arrow technique to identify an idea he conceptualizes as a core belief. He gently tests its strength, breadth, and modifiability and decides not to pursue further evaluation at this time. However, he labels it as an "idea" (implying it is not necessarily a truth) and marks it as a future topic.

PRESENTING CORE BELIEFS

When the therapist believes he has collected sufficient data to hypothesize about the core belief, and when he believes the patient will be sufficiently receptive, he tentatively poses his conceptualization to her.

T: Sally, we've talked about a number of different problems in the past few weeks—your schoolwork, decisions about how to spend the summer, your volunteer job. It sounds as if behind all these problems is an idea you have about yourself, that you're inadequate. Is that right?

P: Yeah. I think so.

Or he might review with the patient a number of related automatic thoughts she had in a variety of situations, and then ask the patient to draw a conclusion as to an underlying theme ("Sally, do you see a common theme in these automatic thoughts?").

With certain patients the therapist uses the Case Conceptualization Diagram (see Chapter 10, Figure 10.1) early in therapy. Either with or without the diagram, he might briefly explore childhood precursors.

T: Do you remember feeling inadequate like this at other times in your life, too? As a child?

P: Yeah, a lot. I remember never being able to do things my brother could.

T: Can you give me some examples?

Obtaining historical data aids the therapist at a later date when he hypothesizes to the patient how she came to believe a core belief and explains how it could be untrue or mostly untrue even though she currently believes it so strongly.

EDUCATING THE PATIENT ABOUT CORE BELIEFS AND MONITORING THEIR OPERATION

It is important for the patient to understand the following about her core belief:

- That it is an idea, not necessarily a truth.
- That she can believe it quite strongly, even "feel" it to be true, and yet have it be mostly or entirely untrue.
- That, as an idea, it can be tested.
- That it is rooted in childhood events; that it may or may not have been true at the time she first came to believe it.
- That it continues to be maintained through the operation of her schemas, in which she readily recognizes data that support the core belief while ignoring or discounting data to the contrary.
- That she and the therapist working together can use a variety of strategies over time to change this idea so that she can view herself in a more realistic way.

In the transcript that follows, the therapist educates Sally about her core belief. (She had previously confirmed the conceptualization he had presented.)

T: Sally, does this [her automatic thought that she will not be able to write her economics paper] sound familiar? Do you think your idea that you're inadequate could be getting in the way?

P: Yeah. I do feel inadequate.

T: Well, Sally, one of two things has been going on. The problem is either you really *are* inadequate, and we'll have to do some work together to make you more adequate . . . or, the problem is that you *believe* you are inadequate; and sometimes, you believe it so strongly that you actually *act* in an inadequate way, like not going to the library to start researching your paper. What do you think?

P: I don't know.

T: Why don't we have you write these two possibilities on paper? This is what I'd like to start doing in therapy, if it is okay with you, seeing which possibility seems more true—that you really *are* inadequate or that you *believe* you're inadequate.

Later in this session or in another session, the therapist explains core beliefs to Sally, in small parts, making sure she understands as he proceeds.

T: This idea, "I'm inadequate," is what we call a core belief. Let me tell you a little bit about core beliefs so you'll understand why they're more difficult to evaluate and respond to. First of all, a core belief is an idea that you may not believe very strongly when you're not depressed. On the other hand, we'd expect you to believe it almost completely when you *are* depressed, even if there's evidence to the contrary. Follow me so far?

P: Yes.

T: When you get depressed, this idea becomes activated. When it's activated, you'll easily notice any evidence that seems to support it and you'll tend to ignore any evidence that contradicts it. It's as if there is a screen around your head. Anything that fits in with the idea that you are inadequate sails straight through the screen and into your head. Any information that contradicts the idea won't fit through the screen and so either you don't notice it, or you change it in some way so it *will* fit through the screen. Do you think you might be screening information like this?

P: I'm not sure.

T: Well, let's see. Looking back at the past few weeks, what evidence is there that you *might* be adequate?

P: Ummm . . . I got an A– on my statistics exam.

T: Good! And did that evidence go right through the screen? Did you tell yourself, "I got an A–; that means I'm smart or adequate or a good student," or anything like that?

P: No. I said, "Well, the exam was easy. I learned some of that stuff last year."

T: Oh, so it looks like the screen *was* operating. Do you see how you discounted information that contradicted your core belief, "I am inadequate"?

P: Hmmm.

T: Can you think of any other examples from this week? Situations where a reasonable person might think something you did showed you were adequate, even if you didn't?

P: (*Thinks for a moment.*) Well, I helped my roommate figure out how to solve a problem with her father. But, that doesn't count; anyone could have done what I did.

T: Good example. Again, it sounds as if you didn't recognize information that doesn't fit in with "I'm inadequate." I'm going to let you think about how true the idea is that anyone could have done what you did. Maybe this is another instance of not giving yourself credit when another person might have thought it was evidence that you are *not* inadequate.

P: Well, my roommate did think I helped her a lot.

T: Okay, just to summarize, "I'm inadequate" seems to be a core belief which goes back a long time with you and which you believe much more strongly when you're depressed. Can you summarize how it seems to work?

P: Well, you're saying that when I'm depressed, I screen in information that agrees with it and I screen out information that doesn't agree with it.

T: Right. How about for homework this week if you try to notice each day how the screen is operating—jot down information that seems to support the idea that you're inadequate. And here's the harder part. Really hunt for and jot down any information that another person might think contradicts it. Okay?

In the next session, the therapist explains why Sally believes her core belief so strongly and how it could still be untrue.

T: Okay, you did a good job this week noticing how you tend to let in only the negative information which seems to support your idea that you're inadequate. As we predicted, it was much harder to recognize positive information that contradicts your idea.

P: Yeah. I didn't do it very well.

T: Are you feeling inadequate now?

P: (*Laughs.*) Yes. I guess so.

T: Is the screen operating right now? Did you put more emphasis on the part of the homework you didn't do as well and forget about the part you did do well?

P: I guess I did.

T: What do you think is the effect of having a screen like this?

P: Makes me not notice the good things.

T: Right. And, day after day, what happens to this idea, "I'm inadequate"?

P: Gets stronger, I guess.

T: Right. To the point where it "feels" true, even if it's not.

P: Hmmm.

T: Do you see now how the idea that you're inadequate *could* be false even though it feels so true?

P: Well, I can kind of see it intellectually, but I still do *feel* inadequate.

T: That's pretty common. In the next few weeks, we'll keep on evaluating this idea. And then we'll work together on helping the more reasonable, rational part of your mind talk to the more emotional side. Okay?

P: Yeah.

Bibliotherapy can reinforce the important core belief work of therapy. Two books in particular, *Prisoners of Belief* (McKay & Fanning, 1991) and *Reinventing Your Life* (Young & Klosko, 1994), are helpful in this phase of therapy.

MODIFYING CORE BELIEFS AND STRENGTHENING NEW BELIEFS

Having identified the negative core belief, the therapist mentally devises a new, more realistic and functional belief and guides the patient toward it. He may use some of the techniques listed on the left side of Figure 11.2 to start attenuating the old belief. Fairly soon, he and the patient collaboratively develop a new, more adaptive belief. A relatively positive belief is generally easier for a patient to adopt than a belief that is at an extreme.

For example:

Old core belief	New core belief
I'm (completely) unlovable.	I'm generally a likable person.
I'm bad.	I'm a worthwhile person with positive and negative features.
I'm powerless.	I have control over many things.
I'm defective.	I'm normal, with both strengths and weaknesses.

Already described	**Additional techniques**
Socratic questioning techniques	Core Belief Worksheet
Examining advantages and disadvantages	Extreme contrasts
Rational–emotional role-play	Developing metaphors
Acting "as if"	Historical tests
Behavioral experiments	Restructuring early memories
Cognitive continuum	Coping cards (see Chapter 12)
Self-disclosure	

FIGURE 11.2. Techniques to modify core beliefs.

The Axis I patient may have believed the "new" core belief during much of her life, and thus it is relatively easy to specify. The Axis II patient, in contrast, may have never had a positive core belief. Therefore, the therapist may need to help her develop an alternative positive core belief. Sally's therapist finds it easy to help her put a more positive core belief into words:

T: Sally, we've been talking about this core belief, "I'm inadequate." What do you rationally think a more accurate belief might be?

P: I am adequate?

T: That's good. Or we could work on a new belief that might be easier for you to adopt, say, "I'm adequate in most ways, but I'm only human, too." Which sounds better?

P: The second.

THE CORE BELIEF WORKSHEET

Having identified the old core belief and developed a new one, the therapist may introduce the Core Belief Worksheet (CBW) (see Figure 11.3). As mentioned previously, it is preferable to introduce this tool after the patient has learned that some of her ideas (automatic thoughts) have been inaccurate or distorted in some way. In addition, core belief work is usually started after the patient has successfully learned the process of evaluating and modifying her automatic thoughts, truly understands that she can modify her dysfunctional thinking, and has established a firm therapeutic alliance with her therapist.

CORE BELIEF WORKSHEET

Old core belief: *I'm inadequate*

How much do you believe the old core belief right now?(0–100) 60%
    *What's the most you've believed it this week?(0–100) 90%
    *What's the least you've believed it this week?(0–100) 60%
New belief: *I'm adequate in most ways (but I'm only human, too).*
How much do you believe the new belief right now?(0–100) 50%

Evidence that contradicts old core belief and supports new belief	Evidence that supports old core belief with reframe
Did good work on literature paper	*Didn't understand econ concept in class BUT I hadn't read about it and I'll probably understand it later. At worst it's an inadequacy but maybe it's actually her fault for not explaining it well enough.*
Asked a question in statistics	
Understand this worksheet	
Got a B on chemistry test	*Didn't go to the teaching assistant for help BUT that doesn't mean I'm inadequate. I was nervous about going because I think I should be able to figure out these things myself and I thought he'd think I was unprepared.*
Made decisions about next year	
Arranged to switch phones, bank accounts, insurance, etc.	
Got together all the references I need for econ paper	*Got a B on my literature paper, BUT it's an okay grade. If I were really inadequate, I wouldn't even be in college.*
Understood most of Chapter 6 in statistics book	
Explained statistics concept to guy down the hall	

*Should situations related to an increase or decrease in the strength of the belief be topics for the agenda?

FIGURE 11.3. Sally's Core Belief Worksheet. Copyright 1993 by Judith S. Beck, Ph.D.

The CBW has two parts: the top part guides the patient to identify and rate her degree of belief in the "old" dysfunctional belief and in the "new," more adaptive belief. Therapist and patient fill out this part together at the beginning of each session following the introduction of the CBW. The bottom part is to be filled out by the patient, both in session and for homework, as she monitors the operation of her beliefs and reframes evidence that seemed to support the old belief.

T: Sally, let me show you a Core Belief Worksheet, which is just an organized way of working on your beliefs. Here, let's write your core belief, "I'm inadequate," at the top. How much do you believe that right now?

P: Maybe 60%.

T: Okay, write "60%" under it. Now, for the next two lines, think about this past week. What's the most and least you've believed it?

P: Most? When I started studying for my statistics exam. Ninety percent, I guess. And least? Now, 60%. (*Writes it down.*)

T: Last week we talked about a more adaptive, not to mention more accurate, belief. Do you remember how we phrased it?

P: Yes. I am adequate in most ways but I am only human, too.

T: Good. Write that under new belief. How much do you believe this new belief today?

P: Maybe . . . 50%.

T: Okay, Sally, we can fill out these ratings every week together at the beginning of our sessions, or you can fill them out just beforehand. I'd like you to keep this sheet in front of you during our sessions to see if the topic we're discussing is relevant to the idea, "I'm inadequate," or not.

P: Okay.

T: Let's start filling out the bottom part now, together, so you can learn how to do it, if that's okay with you. Then, if it's helpful, you can add to it every day.

P: Okay.

T: One more thing. Learning to fill out this sheet takes time and practice, just as it took you a while to get good at the Dysfunctional Thought Record. Okay?

P: Sure.

T: All right. Is it okay if we start with the right side, evidence that you're inadequate?

P: Sure.

T: Okay, think over what you did *today*. What evidence do you have that you're inadequate?

P: Well, I didn't understand a concept my economics professor presented in class today.

T: Okay, write that down on the right side, then put a big "BUT" next to it. . . . Now, let's think if there could be another explanation for why you might not have understood the concept *other* than that you're inadequate.

P: Well, it was the first time she talked about it. And it wasn't in the readings.

T: Good. Now might you be able to grasp it after she has reviewed it, or you've read something about it, or asked someone else to explain it better?

P: Probably.

T: Okay. Now next to the "BUT" you'll write what we call the "reframe"— another, more adaptive way of looking at the evidence. What could you say here?

P: I guess I could say, "But I hadn't read about it, and I'll probably understand it later."

T: Okay, write that down. . . . Now let's see if we can make the reframe even stronger. Would you agree that not understanding a concept at worst means a person has *an* inadequacy, not that she's completely inadequate as a person?

P: Yes, that's true.

T: Is it possible that *many* adequate people don't necessarily grasp concepts at the first presentation?

P: True.

T: I wonder, is it possible that it was actually an inadequacy of the *professor*, because if she had explained it more clearly, more people might have understood it?

P: That's possible.

T: Why don't you take a minute and see if there is anything else you want to add in writing. . . . Okay, let's try the left side now. What evidence do you have from *today* that you *are* adequate at many things? I'll warn you, this can be hard if your screen is operating.

P: Well, I worked on my literature paper.

T: Good. Write that down. What else?

P: I asked a question in my statistics course.

T: You did! Good. What else?

P: (*No response.*)

T: How about the fact that you seem to grasp how to do this worksheet?

P: I guess so.

T: Okay, how about for homework if you try to add to the bottom of this sheet every day. Can you see that to start, doing the first part of the right side will be easiest, but the second part and the left side will probably be harder?

P: Yeah.

T: So do what you can. It may be that we'll have to work together to do the reframes and look for positive evidence. I'll give you a clue, though. If you have trouble with these two parts, pretend someone else, your roommate, for example, has done exactly what you've done, and see how you'd view her actions. Okay?

P: Sure.

T: Can you think of anything that might get in the way of your doing this assignment this week?

P: No, I'll try it.

T: Good.

Had Sally displayed difficulty in identifying any positive data during the session, her therapist would have postponed this homework assignment, trying different techniques in session first to help her successfully elicit items for the left side. For example, he might use a contrasting technique:

T: How about the fact that you battled your way through the student health system so you would get seen right away? Doesn't that belong on the left side?

P: I don't know. I was just so mad; it was easy.

T: Wait a minute. If you *hadn't* asserted yourself, wouldn't you have put that on the right side as a sign of inadequacy?

P: Probably.

T: So think of it this way. Anything that you would criticize yourself for or put on the right side if you *didn't* do it, probably belongs on the left.

Other ways of having the patient recognize positive data that belong on the left side of the worksheet include:

1. [As in the transcript on p. 180,] asking the patient to think of data that she would say were positive evidence for *another* person: "Sally, can you think of someone else who you consider is adequate in most ways? Who would that be? What have *you* done today that you would say shows that Donna is adequate if *she* had done it?"

2. Asking the patient to think of data that *someone else* would probably say indicate positive evidence for the patient: "Sally, who's someone you think knows you pretty well, whose judgment you trust? What would [this person] say you had done today that's evidence you're adequate?" or "Sally, what have you done today that *I* probably think indicates you're adequate?"

3. Asking the patient to reflect on whether she would discount specific positive evidence if she compared what she did to a hypothetical *negative* model: "Sally, you don't believe that finishing that brief paper is a sign of adequacy. But would a *truly* inadequate person have been able to write it? Would a truly inadequate person even have made it to where you are now?"

4. Asking the patient to fill out the ratings at the top of the CBW (with a previously agreed-on core belief filled in) at the beginning of each session, before setting the agenda. Then the therapist can ask, "When you believed *least* strongly that you were inadequate, what was going on? Is this something we should put on the agenda?" Discussion of these (more positive) situations provides an opportunity to gather or reinforce evidence for the left side. (Note that the CBW has reminders of these questions printed at the bottom.)

The therapist may also take the opportunity throughout the session to question the patient about the applicability of the CBW to the topic at hand.

T: Sally, can you summarize what we've just been talking about?

P: Well, I was pretty down because I didn't get the summer job I wanted, and where anyone would probably be disappointed, I got pretty depressed because what it meant to me was that I was inadequate.

T: Good. Can you see how this is relevant to the Core Belief Worksheet?

P: Yeah. It's the same idea.

T: How can you write it down on the worksheet?

P: I guess it goes on the *right side.* . . . I didn't get the research assistant job . . . but that doesn't mean I'm completely inadequate. A lot of people applied for it, some with lots more experience than me.

Using Extreme Contrasts to Modify Core Beliefs

At times, it is helpful for patients to compare themselves with someone, either real or imagined, who is at a negative extreme of the quality related to the patient's core belief. The therapist suggests that the patient imagine someone within her frame of reference. (This technique is similar to the cognitive continuum described in Chapter 12.)

T: I wonder, do you know anyone at your school who truly *is* inadequate or at least *behaves* very inadequately?

P: Ummm . . . There is one guy in my dorm who never, I think, goes to classes or does work. He just seems to party all the time. I think he's failing.

T: Okay, so compared to him, how inadequate are you?

P: (*Pauses.*) Not very.

T: If you truly were an inadequate person, through and through, what would you be doing differently?

P: . . . I guess I'd drop out of college, sit around all day . . . not support myself . . . not do anything worthwhile . . . not have any friends—

T: How close are you to that now?

P: Not at all, I guess.

T: So how accurate would you say it is to label yourself as truly inadequate?

P: I guess it's really not accurate.

Developing Metaphors

Therapists can help patients distance themselves from core beliefs by reflecting on a different situation. One patient believed she must be bad because as a child (and as an adult) her mother treated her so badly. It was helpful for her to reflect on the story of Cinderella, in which a wicked stepmother treats a child quite badly without the child's being at fault or being bad.

Historical Tests of the Core Belief

It is often useful to have the patient examine how a belief originated and became maintained through the years (Young, 1990). The therapist helps the patient to search for (and reframe) evidence that seemed to support the core belief from an early age and also to uncover evidence that contradicted it. (The CBW can be used for such a process.) Usually, this process is initiated after the patient has been monitoring the operation of her core belief in the *present* and has started the process of modifying it, via the CBW or other techniques.

It is not always necessary for the patient to have a strong activation of her core belief for this process to be effective, though some patients may not have access to some important memories unless they are emotionally aroused with an activated core belief. The therapist first provides a rationale.

T: Sally, I'd like to see where this idea that you're inadequate started.

P: Okay.

T: Let's pull out the Core Belief Worksheet and work forward in time. Do you remember anything when you were quite young that made you believe at the time that you were inadequate? Say, before elementary school?

P: I remember nursery school. I remember doing something with puzzles and the teacher yelling at me. I was crying and crying—

T: Were you slow to finish it?

P: Yes, something like that.

T: And you felt pretty inadequate?

P: Uh huh.

T: Okay, write that down on the right-hand side. We'll fill in the reframes later. What else?

P: I remember this time my family went to Valley Forge State Park. And everyone else could ride their bikes around, but I couldn't keep up, and I got left really far behind.

Either in session, or for homework, the patient continues this first step: recording memories that may have contributed to the core belief. She may reflect on preschool, elementary school, high school, college, her 20's, 30's, etc. The second step of the historical review involves searching for and recording evidence that supports the new, positive belief for each period. Having evoked more positive memories, the patient is ready for the third step: reframing each piece of negative evidence. Finally, in the fourth step, the patient summarizes each period. For example:

> *High School Years*—I did a lot of things competently, from sports to being responsible for a lot of things at home to doing well at school. It's true that I didn't get all A's, and I wasn't good at everything, and I *felt* inadequate at times, but basically I was adequate.

Restructuring Early Memories

For many Axis I patients, the "rational" or "intellectual" techniques that have already been presented are sufficient to modify a core belief. For others, special "emotional" or experiential techniques, in which the patient's affect is aroused, are also indicated. One such technique involves role-playing, reenacting an event to help the patient reinterpret an earlier, traumatic experience. In the transcript that follows, the therapist helps the patient restructure the meaning of an earlier event related to a current distressing situation.

T: Sally, you look pretty down today.

P: Yes. (*Crying.*) . . . I got my paper back. I got a C–. I can't do anything right.

T: Are you feeling pretty inadequate?

P: Yes.

T: (*Heightening her affect to facilitate memory retrieval.*) Do you feel this sadness and inadequacy somewhere in your body?

P: Behind my eyes. And my shoulders feel heavy.

T: When is the first time you remember feeling this way, as a kid?

P: (*Pause.*) When I was 6 or 7. I remember I brought home my report card, and I was a little scared because I hadn't done very well. My dad was okay about it, but my mom got pretty mad.

T: What did she say?

P: She yelled, "Sally, what am I going to do with you! Just look at this report card!"

T: What did you say?

P: I don't think I said anything. But that just made her madder. She kept saying, "Don't you know what will happen if you don't get good grades? Your brother always does well. Why can't you? I'm so ashamed of you. What are you going to amount to?"

T: You must have felt pretty bad.

P: I did.

T: Do you think this was a reasonable way for her to act?

P: No . . . I guess not.

T: Well, is this something you'd say to your own kids some day?

P: No. I'd never say that.

T: What would *you* say if you had a 7-year-old daughter who brought home a report card like that?

P: Ummm . . . I guess I'd say what my father did, "That's okay. Don't feel bad. I didn't do great in school either and it didn't matter one bit."

T: That's good. Do you have any idea why your mother didn't say that?

P: I'm not sure.

T: I wonder, from what you've told me before, if it could be because she thought other people might look down on *her* if her kids didn't do well.

P: That's probably right. She was always bragging about my brother to her friends. I think she was always trying to keep up with the Joneses.

T: Okay, how about if we do a role-play. I'll play you at age 7; you play your mom. Try to see things from her point of view as much as you can. I'll start. . . . Mom, here's my report card.

P: Sally, I'm ashamed of you. Look at these grades. What am I going to do with you?

T: Mom, I'm only 7. My grades aren't great like Robert's, but they're okay.

P: Don't you know what will happen if you don't get good grades? You'll never amount to anything.

T: That's silly, Mom. I'm only 7.

P: But next year, you will be 8, and after that 9—

T: Mom, I didn't do that bad. Why are you making such a big deal? You're making me feel like I'm completely inadequate. Is that what you mean to do?

P: No, of course not. I don't want you to think that. It's not true. I just want you to do better.

T: Okay, out of role. What do you think?

P: I wasn't really inadequate. I did okay. Mom probably was hard on me because *she* didn't want to be criticized. (*Brightens.*)

T: How much do you believe that?

P: A lot. 80%.

T: How about if we do the role-play again, but this time we'll switch parts. Let's see how well the 7-year-old Sally can talk back to her mother.

Following this second role-play, the therapist asks Sally what she learned and how this learning applies to the situation which upset her this week (getting a C– on a paper).

Another technique uses imagery to restructure early memories in the presence of affect (Edwards, 1989; Layden et al., 1993). This Gestalt therapy type of technique has been adapted specifically to change core beliefs and is more often used with patients with personality disorders than with Axis I patients. Again, the therapist has the patient reexperience an early distressing event that seems to have helped originate or maintain a core belief. The following extended case example illustrates how the therapist does the following:

1. Identifies a specific situation that is currently quite distressing to the patient and seems linked to an important core belief;
2. Heightens the patient's affect by focusing on automatic thoughts, emotions, and somatic sensations;
3. Helps the patient identify and reexperience a relevant early experience;
4. Talks to the "younger" part of the patient to identify automatic thoughts, emotions, and beliefs; and
5. Helps the patient develop a different understanding of the experience through guided imagery, Socratic questioning, dialogue, and/or role-play.

In the following transcript, Sally reports an upsetting experience from the previous day in which she felt criticized by her study group.

T: Can you imagine this scene again, as if it's happening right now? You're all sitting around the table—

[Therapist has Sally vividly picture and describe the distressing incident.]

P: Peggy is saying, "Sally, you didn't do this thoroughly enough. You'll have to beef it up." And I'm feeling so down, so sad. [I'm thinking] "I'm letting everyone down. I'm not good enough. I can't do anything right. I'll probably flunk out."

T: Are you feeling the sadness right now?

P: (*Nods.*)

T: Where in your body do you feel it?

P: Behind my eyes.

T: Anywhere else? Where else is the sadness?

P: In my chest . . . and my stomach. There's a heaviness.

T: Okay, can you focus on the heaviness? Can you really feel it now, in your stomach, in your chest? And behind your eyes?

P: (*Nods.*)

T: Okay, just focus on your eyes, your stomach, your chest. . . . (*Waits about 10 seconds.*) Sally, when do you remember feeling this heaviness before, when you were a kid? When's the *first* time you remember feeling like this?

In the next section, the therapist has Sally reexperience a distressing, significant memory and interviews the "child" part of Sally to identify what sense she had made of this early experience at the time. (Note that the therapist continually reinforces the emotional immediacy of the experience by having the patient use the present tense throughout.)

P: . . . My mom. My mom is yelling at me.

T: How old are you, Sally?

P: About 6 or 7. I'm not sure.

T: Where are you? Describe it for me as vividly as you can.

P: I'm home. I'm doing my homework. I have to do some kind of worksheet. I can't do it. I have to mark long and short vowels or something. I don't know what to do. I've been absent. I don't know how to do this.

T: What happens next?

P: Mom walks in the kitchen: "Get to bed, Sally." "I can't. I have to finish my homework. . . ."

T: And then?

P: She says, "You've been at this forever. I told you half an hour ago to go to bed."

T: What do you say?

P: "But I have to do this. I'll get in trouble."

T: And then?

P: She says, "What's the matter with you? Why can't you finish this? It's easy. What are you, stupid? Get in bed, now!"

T: And then?

P: I run to my room.

T: And then?

P: I don't know. Go to sleep, I guess. (*Looks down, very sad.*)

T: When is the worst point?

P: When she's yelling at me.

T: Okay, can you picture this again? Where are you?

P: I'm sitting at the kitchen table.

T: And you're struggling with your homework? You don't know what to do?

P: Yeah.

T: And your mom comes into the kitchen? How does she look? Where is she?

P: She's tall. Standing up. She looks mad.

T: How can you tell?

P: (*Eyes begin to tear.*) Her face is scrunched up. Her body looks tense.

T: And she says . . . ?

P: "Sally, go to bed."

T: Keep going.

P: "Mom, I can't. I have to finish this." "I said, Get to bed! What's the matter with you? This stuff is easy. Are you stupid?" (*Sobs.*)

T: (*Gently.*) Six-year-old Sally, how are you feeling?

P: Sad. (*Cries a little.*)

T: Real sad?

P: (*Nods.*)

T: (*Softly.*) Six-year-old Sally, what's going through your mind right now?

P: I *am* stupid. I can't do anything right.

T: How much do you believe that?

P: Completely.

T: Anything else going through your mind?

P: I'll never be able to do stuff right.

Note that the intensification of affect in the experience is the clue that verifies that this is a core issue for this patient. In the next section, the therapist helps Sally reinterpret this experience.

T: Six-year-old Sally, I'd like to help you see this a different way. What do you think would help? Would you like to talk to your mom, explain to her why you're having a hard time? Or, would you like someone to explain to *you* what's going on . . . your 18-year-old self, maybe? Or someone else? How can we get you to see this a different way, 6-year-old Sally?

P: I don't want to talk to Mom. She'll just yell at me.

T: Would you like your older self to explain it to you, 6-year-old Sally?

P: Yes.

T: Okay, can you imagine that your mom walks out of the kitchen and your 18-year-old self walks in? Where would you like her to be?

P: Next to me, I guess.

T: Real close?

P: (*Nods.*)

T: Would you like her to put her arm around you?

P: (*Nods.*)

T: Okay. Let's have 18-year-old Sally talk to 6-year-old Sally. Have her ask 6-year-old Sally what's wrong.

P: "What's wrong?" "I feel so stupid. I can't do anything right."

T: What does your older self answer back?

P: "No, you're not. This homework is too hard. It's not your fault. You're not stupid."

T: What does 6-year-old Sally say?

P: "But I should be able to do it."

T: Have your older self keep talking to her.

P: "No, that's not true. You shouldn't be able to do it. You've been absent. You were never taught this. Actually, it's your teacher's fault for giving you something too hard."

T: Does 6-year-old Sally believe her?

P: A little.

T: What does 6-year-old Sally want to ask?

P: "Why does everything have to be so hard? Why can't I do anything right?"

T: What does the older Sally say?

P: "You do lots of things right. Some things like math papers are easy, and getting dressed all by yourself and playing baseball. . . ."

T: What is 6-year-old Sally thinking?

P: "But I can't play baseball well. Robert is so much better."

T: What does your older self say to that?

P: "Listen, he *is* better at baseball than you. But he's *older*. When he was your age, he could only do what you can do now. You'll get better, just wait."

T: How is 6-year-old Sally feeling now?

When the patient reports that her younger self is feeling significantly less sad, the therapist wraps up the exercise (e.g., "Is there anything else you want to ask your older self, 6-year-old Sally?"). If the patient reports that she is still quite upset, he might try another tack; for example:

T: Let me talk to 6-year-old Sally for a minute. Six-year-old Sally, you're still so sad. Why do you *still* think you can't do anything right?

P: (*Thinks.*) Mom. She tells me so. She's right.

T: Would you like to try to talk to her?

P: (*Reluctantly.*) I'm not sure.

T: How about if we do a role-play? Six-year-old Sally, you be your mother. I'll be you. You start. Pretend you're coming in the kitchen and you see me doing my homework.

P: Okay . . . Sally, get to bed. Now!

T: But, Mom, I have to finish my homework or I'll get in trouble.

P: What's the matter with you? You must be stupid.

T: No, I'm not, Mom. The teacher made a mistake. This worksheet is too hard.

P: If it's too hard, there must be something wrong with you.

T: No, Mom. That's not true. Mom, do you really think there's something wrong with me? Do you want me to grow up thinking I'm stupid and can't do anything right?

P: (*Pauses.*) No . . . no. I don't think you're stupid. I don't want you to grow up thinking that.

T: Then why did you call me stupid if it's not true?

P: I shouldn't have. It's not true.

T: Why did you?

P: (*Pauses.*) I don't know. I just get so frustrated sometimes. I really just want you in bed so I can have some peace and quiet.

T: You mean you don't think I'm stupid?

P: No . . . no. I don't. You're not stupid.

T: But there are so many things I can't do. I can't read very well. I can't even ride a two-wheeler bike. Robert can do those things.

P: But he's older. You'll be able to do them someday, too.

T: But you yell at me a lot for not doing things well. You yelled at me about this worksheet. You're always yelling at me about not cleaning my room well enough or not doing the dishes well enough or not getting good enough marks on tests.

P: I do expect a lot from you. I don't know. Maybe too much, sometimes. But that's my job. I'm supposed to push you. How will you grow up if I don't?

T: Mom, your pushing me makes me feel like I'm inadequate and stupid and like I can't do anything right. Is that what you want me to grow up believing?

P: No, of course not.

T: What *do* you want me to believe?

P: That you're smart, that you can do whatever you want to.

T: Do you believe that, Mom? That I'm smart and can do anything I want?

P: Yes, I do. I'm sorry.

T: Okay. Out of role-play for the moment. Now how are you feeling?

P: Better.

T: Let's do the role-play again. This time you play 6-year-old Sally, sitting at the kitchen table, struggling with her homework. Pay close attention to how she's feeling and what she's thinking. Let's start. I'm Mom, and I walk into the kitchen and I say, "Sally, get to bed. Now!"

Sally and the therapist continue the role-play to give Sally the opportunity to test the validity of her thoughts and conclusions with her mother. At the end, the therapist asks Sally to write down the old belief that was activated in this memory and the new belief and to rate how much she now believes each one. Then they discuss the present distressing incident involving her friend Peggy and the study group and help Sally draw a more reality-based, more adaptive conclusion. By the end of the session, Sally believes only 20% that she is inadequate and 70% that she is adequate. She believes an alternative explanation quite strongly: that her contribution may not live up to Peggy's expectations, but that does not make it completely inadequate; that even if it is not as good as it could be does not mean *she* is completely inadequate as a person; and that the major reason for its lack of breadth was the study group's lack of specified guidelines and Sally's relative inexperience working in a study group.

In summary, core beliefs require consistent, systematic work. A number of techniques, applicable to restructuring automatic thoughts and intermediate beliefs, may be used along with more specialized techniques oriented specifically toward core beliefs.

Chapter 12

ADDITIONAL COGNITIVE AND BEHAVIORAL TECHNIQUES

A number of cognitive and behavioral techniques have been pre viously introduced, among them Socratic questioning, rational–emotional role-playing, Core Belief Worksheets, imagery, and listing advantages and disadvantages of beliefs. This chapter describes other equally important techniques, many of which are both cognitive and behavioral in nature. As described more fully in Chapter 16, the therapist chooses a technique according to his overall conceptualization and his goals for a particular session.

The techniques described in this chapter, as is the case for all cognitive therapy techniques, aim to influence the patient's thinking, behavior, and mood. They include problem-solving, making decisions, behavioral experiments, activity monitoring and scheduling, distraction and refocusing, relaxation techniques, coping cards, graded exposure, role-play, the "pie" technique, functional comparisons of oneself, and positive self-statement logs. Additional techniques are described in various sources (Beck & Emery, 1985; McMullin, 1986).

PROBLEM-SOLVING

Associated with or in addition to their psychological disorders, patients have real-life problems. The therapist inquires about such problems in the first session, creating a "problem list" or translating each problem into positive goals (Chapter 3). At every session, he encourages the patient to put on the agenda problems that have come up during the week or problems she anticipates might arise in the coming weeks. While the therapist might take a more active role initially in suggesting possible solutions, he encourages the patient to do active problem-solving herself as therapy progresses.

Some patients are deficient in problem-solving skills. They often

193

benefit from direct instruction in problem-solving, where they learn to specify a problem, devise solutions, select a solution, implement it, and evaluate its effectiveness. Many patients, however, already possess good problem-solving skills. They need help in testing dysfunctional beliefs that impede problem-solving.

Sally, for example, had difficulty concentrating when she was studying. Her therapist suggested several practical ideas for her to try: starting with the easiest assignment first, reviewing relevant class notes before reading the textbook, writing down questions when she was unsure of her understanding, and pausing every few minutes to rehearse mentally what she had just read. They agreed she would try these strategies as experiments to see which, if any, facilitated her concentration and comprehension.

Another problem arose several sessions later. Sally had started a volunteer job tutoring a neighborhood child. Although the child was cooperative, Sally felt unsure of what she was doing. Intellectually she knew how to solve the problem; she realized she should contact the agency that coordinated the volunteers and/or the child's teacher. Her belief that she should not ask for help, however, inhibited her. After evaluating her automatic thoughts and beliefs about this specific situation, Sally implemented the solution she herself had initially conceived.

Another problem arose when Sally had to write a term paper for a course. Her therapist used a Problem-Solving Worksheet (see Figure 12.1) along with Socratic questioning to help Sally identify and respond to a dysfunctional belief which promoted her procrastination.

Some problem-solving may involve significant life changes. After careful evaluation of a situation, a therapist might encourage a battered spouse to seek refuge or take legal action. A patient chronically dissatisfied with her job might be helped to analyze the advantages and disadvantages of the job. If the disadvantages are stronger and/or more numerous, her therapist might discuss finding a new job or training for a different career. A patient in an unsatisfying relationship or living situation might first choose, with the therapist's help, to investigate improving the status quo; if insufficient progress is made, she may then choose to change her situation.

DECISION-MAKING

Common to many patients is difficulty making a decision. The therapist asks the patient to list the advantages and disadvantages of each choice and then helps her devise a system for weighing each item and drawing a conclusion about which option seems best. (See Figure 12.2.)

PROBLEM-SOLVING WORKSHEET

Patient's name: _Sally_   Date: _4/12_

(When automatic thoughts, beliefs, and/or high emotions interfere with straightforward problem-solving)

1. Problem

   Starting paper for economics course.

2. Special meaning: automatic thoughts and beliefs

   I'm not competent enough to do it.

3. Response to special meaning

   I'm competent enough to turn in something. I don't actually know how well I'll do 'til I do it.

4. Possible solution(s)

   1. *Stick with original idea.*
   2. *Jot down outline on paper (1/2 hour).*
   3. *Talk about ideas to roommate.*
   4. *Read suggested readings and take brief notes.*
   5. *Write first draft; try for a C job, not an A job.*

FIGURE 12.1. Problem-Solving Worksheet. Copyright 1993 by Judith S. Beck, Ph.D.

THERAPIST: You mentioned that you wanted help in deciding whether to go to summer school or to get a job?

PATIENT: Yes.

T: Okay. (*Pulls out a piece of paper.*) Let me show you how to weigh advantages and disadvantages. Have you ever done that?

P: No. At least not in writing. I've been going over some of the pros and cons in my head.

T: Good. That'll help us get started. I think you'll find that writing them down will make the decision clearer. Which one do you want to start with—school or a job?

P: Getting a job, I guess.

T: Okay. Write "Advantages of job" at the top left of this paper and "Disadvantages of job" on the top right and "Advantages of school" and "Disadvantages of school" at the bottom.

P: (*Does so.*) Okay.

Advantages of job	**Disadvantages of job**
1. Make money.	1. Have to find one.
2. Maybe learn skills.	2. Less free time.
3. Break from what I've been doing.	3. Might not like it.
4. Meet different people.	
5. Make me feel more productive.	
6. Good for resume.	

Advantages of summer school	**Disadvantages of summer school**
1. Two friends are going.	1. Not making money and it costs money.
2. Could take one less course in the fall.	2. Doesn't increase my skills.
3. Lots of free time.	3. More of the same of what I've been doing.
4. It's a known quantity.	4. Doesn't make me feel as productive.
5. Could meet new people.	5. Doesn't help my resume.
6. Easier to enroll than to find a job.	

FIGURE 12.2. Sally's advantages–disadvantages analysis.

T: What have you been thinking? Could you jot down some advantages and disadvantages of getting a job at the top? (*The patient writes down the ideas she has had so far. The therapist asks some questions to guide her.*) How about the fact that you'd be doing something different—taking a break from schoolwork—is that an advantage?

P: Yeah. (*Writes it down.*)

T: How about that a job might cut into your vacation time?

P: No, I'd only take a job that would let me spend the last 2 weeks of August with my family.

The therapist and patient continue this process until the patient feels she has recorded both sides fairly and thoroughly. They repeat the process with the second option. Examining advantages and disadvantages of summer school reminds the patient of some additional items to add to the "job" lists. Likewise, the patient also reviews the "job" items to see whether their counterparts are relevant to the "summer school" lists.

Next, the therapist helps the patient evaluate the items:

T: Okay, Sally, this looks pretty complete. Now we want you to weigh the items in some way. You could rate how important each one is 0–10. Or, you could circle the most important items. What do you think?

P: Circle the items, I guess.

T: Okay, let's look at the "job" lists. Which are most important to you? (*The patient circles items in each column in Figure 12.2.*) Just looking over what you've circled, what do you think?

P: Seems like the big stumbling block with a summer job is having to *find* one. Because if I had one, I think I *would* like to make money, I would feel more productive, and it would be good to get a break from school.

T: Should we spend a few minutes now talking about how you might go about looking for a job? Then we can come back to this list and see if you're still leaning that way.

At the end of the discussion, the therapist tries to enhance the probability that the patient will use this technique again:

T: Did you find this process of listing and weighing advantages and disadvantages useful? Can you think of any other decisions you might have where it'd be good to do the same thing? How will you remember to do it this way?

BEHAVIORAL EXPERIMENTS

Behavioral experiments directly test the validity of the patient's thoughts or assumptions and are an important evaluative technique, used alone or accompanied by Socratic questioning. These experiments can be done in or out of the office. Here is an example:

T: Okay, so you believe very strongly, 95%, that you can't concentrate well enough to read. Is that just sometimes or all the time?

P: All the time.

T: I wonder if we could test that idea right now. I have today's newspaper. How about taking a look at this article—it made me pretty mad; it's about how they're going to raise our electric bills again. [The therapist chose a short article he believes the patient will understand.]

P: Okay. (*Reads article.*)

T: Finished? What do you think? Should our rates be going up?

P: I'm not sure. [The writer] did make a case for needing to cover the costs of rewiring after the big storm this winter.

T: You may be right. I guess I'm automatically suspicious when a public utility proposes to raise its rates. . . . In any case, what do you think now about your idea that you can't concentrate?

P: I guess I can do better than I thought.

Other automatic thoughts that can be directly tested in the office include:

Automatic thought	Behavioral experiment
I don't know what to say to him.	Patient role-plays herself while therapist plays other part.
I can't [get myself to] call for a doctor's appointment.	Patient makes phone call in the office.
There are no jobs I'm qualified for.	Patient reviews want ads with therapist.
If I get more and more dizzy, I'll pass out.	Patient creates dizziness through hyperventilating while spinning in a chair (Clark, 1989).

Many homework assignments, too, involve behavioral experiments which the therapist carefully helps to set up, as follows:

1. The patient expresses a negative prediction; the therapist proposes she test it during the week.

2. Collaboratively they decide how, when, and where the patient will test it. The therapist suggests changes, if needed, to maximize the likelihood of success.

3. The therapist asks the patient how she will react if the experiment does confirm the patient's fears so they can devise a response in advance.

An example follows:

T: Okay, Sally, you have a thought and an image of being so tongue-tied in class that you won't be able to ask a question. [The therapist questions Sally as described in Chapter 8, weighing the evidence, examining the worst, best and most realistic outcomes, etc. It seems likely that Sally *will* be able to express herself, though perhaps not perfectly.] How would you feel about doing an experiment this week—testing your thought that you can't ask a question?

P: A little nervous. But I could try.

T: Which class would you like to try? Which would be the easiest for the first time?

P: Literature, I guess.

T: Do you have an idea what question you could ask?

P: (*Thinks for a moment.*) There is something I didn't understand. We've been reading a novel about 18th-century England. I don't understand whether it was just the main character's family that treated women as property or whether it was her social class or whether it was all of society at that time.

T: Good question. How could you phrase it to the professor?

P: I don't know. . . . I guess I could say, "Charlotte's family treated her like property. Was that how all of English society felt at that time or just her social class or just her family?"

T: Good. Asking that question will be a good test of your prediction that you'll be too tongue-tied to talk in class. If you do it and it goes well, that's fine. If you find you're too tongue-tied, we'll work more on that problem next session. But meanwhile, let's suppose for a moment that you *do* have some trouble getting the words out. What do you suppose will go through your mind then?

P: That I'm stupid.

T: I guess we'd better prepare you to respond to that thought now so you won't get demoralized. Okay? [The therapist helps Sally evaluate this thought through standard Socratic questioning and composing a coping card.]

Other assumptions Sally tested using a behavioral experiment outside the therapy session included the following:

- If I talk to [a classmate I don't know] before class, she will snub me.
- If I go to a professor, he won't help me.

(*cont.*)

- If I go to the party Saturday night, I'll have a terrible time.
- If I try to read Chapter 12, I won't understand it.
- Even if I start working on a paper, I won't be able to finish it.

Properly set up, behavioral experiments can be powerful agents of cognitive and emotional change.

ACTIVITY MONITORING AND SCHEDULING

An activity chart is simply a chart with days of the week across the top and each hour down the left-hand side. Figure 12.3 shows a partially completed form. This chart can be used in several different ways, including monitoring the patient's activities, measuring and analyzing pleasure and mastery, monitoring and measuring negative moods, scheduling pleasurable activities or overwhelming tasks, and checking predictions.

The therapist may ask a patient first to monitor her activities to collect relevant data. As with any assignment, the therapist first provides a rationale, ensures that the patient agrees with and understands the assignment, starts the assignment in session, and checks for obstacles. Typically this assignment is proposed early in therapy, in the second or third session. The data it provides can be invaluable, and subsequent changes in the patient's activities often improve her mood significantly.

T: From your description, it sounds as if you're having a tough time getting things done and that you're not enjoying yourself much these days. Is that right?

P: Yes.

T: I wonder if it might be worth monitoring your activities on this activity chart so that next week we can see how you're spending your time. And you can rate your activities to see how much pleasure and sense of accomplishment you get from what you do.

P: Okay.

T: Suppose we make up a pleasure scale first so you'll have a guideline to rate your activities. Now on a scale from 0–10, what activity would you call a 10? An activity that has given you the most pleasure or that you could imagine giving you the most pleasure?

P: Oh, I guess that would be getting an A+ on a paper.

T: Okay, write "10 = A+ on paper" on the chart.

P: (*Does so.*)

T: Now, what would you call a 0? An activity that gives you absolutely no pleasure?

P: Studying for the chemistry exam.

T: All right, write "0 = studying for chemistry exam." . . . What would be 5 on your scale?

P: I guess. . . . having dinner with my roommate.

T: Good, write that. . . . Now what would be about a 3 and a 7?

If the patient can easily match activities with numbers, these five anchor points are usually sufficient. The therapist might give the patient the option of filling in the rest of the scale for homework or leaving it as is. If the patient has difficulty measuring degrees of pleasure, the therapist and patient might collaboratively decide the following:

1. To complete the scale in session.
2. To change the scale to "low, medium, and high."
3. To return to this assignment at a later session.

Sometimes patients assign "0" to an activity that does not seem to warrant such an extreme rating. In this case, the therapist might gently question the accuracy of the scale or do some self-disclosure. "So cleaning the bathroom gives you 0 on the pleasure scale. I wonder if there's anything worse? I know fighting with someone or yelling at my kids when they don't deserve it is a 0 for me."

After sufficiently completing the pleasure scale, the patient fills out the accomplishment scale in the same way.

T: Now, let's make a scale for mastery—which is the sense of accomplishment you feel from an activity. What would be a 10?

P: (*Thinks for a moment.*) Figuring out a really difficult problem in chemistry.

T: What would be a 0?

P: No sense of accomplishment? I don't know. Scrubbing the bathroom would be at least a one. Maybe watching a really bad TV movie.

T: What would be a 5?

P: Oh, balancing my checkbook, I guess. (*Patient fills in scale.*)

T: That's good. Now let's have you fill in a little of today's schedule. Here—it's the 11:00 block—write "therapy" and under that, "A = _____" and "P = _____." Now how much of a sense of accomplishment have you felt during therapy today?

ACTIVITY CHART

	Day 1	Day 2	Day 3	Day 4	Day 5	Day 6	Day 7
6–7 am							
7–8							
8–9	Morning routine A = 2 P = 0						
9–10	Studying A = 2 P = 0						
10–11	Therapy A = 5 P = 4						
11–12 noon	Sit outside A = 1 P = 3						
12–1	Lunch A = 1 P = 3						
1–2	Chem class A = 3 P = 3						
2–3	↓						
3–4	Studying A = 2 P = 1						
4–5	↓						
5–6	↓						
6–7	Dinner A = 2 P = 4						
7–8	TV A = 2 P = 2						
8–9	↓						
9–10	↓						
10–11	↓						
11–12 mid	Sleep						
12–1	↓						
1–2	↓						
2–3	↓						
3–4	↓						
4–5	↓						
5–6	↓						

FIGURE 12.3. Activity chart. Copyright 1995 by Judith S. Beck, Ph.D.

Accomplishment Scale		Pleasure Scale		Conclusions
0	Watching a bad TV movie	0	Studying for chem exam	
1		1		
2		2		
3	Cleaning off my desk	3	Riding my bike around campus	
4		4		
5	Balancing my checkbook	5	Having dinner with roommate	
6		6		
7		7		
8	Finishing my English lit paper	8	Winning dorm baseball game	
9		9		
10	Figuring out difficult chem problem	10	Getting A+ on paper	

FIGURE 12.3. *(cont.)*

P: About a 5.

T: And pleasure?

P: About a 4. (*Fills in the blocks.*)

T: And what did you do in the hour right before therapy today?

P: I was studying in the library.

T: Okay. Write "studying in library" in the block before therapy and write "A = _____" and "P = _____." . . . Now, look at the scale. How much of a sense of accomplishment did you get during that hour? And how much of a sense of pleasure?

P: Let's see, my sense of accomplishment was pretty low, 0, I guess.

T: So studying in the library this morning was about the same as watching a bad TV movie?

P: No. I guess I got some sense of accomplishment. It should be about a 2.

T: And the pleasure?

P: It was the same as studying for the chem exam—0.

T: Okay, write down those numbers. [The therapist and patient fill in more blocks below "studying" until the therapist is satisfied that the patient is accurately and easily assessing her activities.] Now, do you think you're straight on what you have to do?

P: Yeah.

T: Could you tell me why it might be worth the effort to do all this?

P: Well, it seems like it might help me get more organized—see where the time is going.

T: And the accomplishment and pleasure ratings?

P: I don't know.

T: Do you think that looking over the whole week we might learn some things? For example, what activities should you be doing more of or less of? What activities did you used to do that were high in pleasure or accomplishment that you're not doing now? What activities are now low in a sense of accomplishment and pleasure that used to be high?

P: Yeah.

T: Now the ideal thing would be to have you fill this out as close to the time you finish an activity as you can—so you won't forget what you did and so your ratings will be more accurate. If that's impossible, could you try to fill this out at lunch, dinner, and bedtime?

P: Yeah, it shouldn't be a problem.

T: And if you can fill it out every day, that would give us the most information. But even if you just do a couple of days, that would give us some. Now, can you think of anything that might get in the way of your doing this? Any practical problems or thoughts?

P: I just may not remember to do it all the time.

T: Can you think of a way so you'll be more likely to remember?

P: Well, I could carry it in my notebook—I'd see it and it would remind me.

T: Any other problems?

P: No, I should be able to do it.

T: Good. Now one last thing. How about if you look over the activity chart the day before or the day of our next session. See if there are any patterns or if you learn anything from it. You can write down your conclusions at the bottom or on the back. Okay?

P: Yeah.

T: How about writing down this assignment on your homework sheet so we'll both have a copy.

P: Okay. (*Writes down assignment.*)

Reviewing the Activity Chart (the Following Week)

Together the therapist and patient review the activity chart, looking for patterns and drawing conclusions. For example:

> 1. Which activities are over-represented in terms of leading a balanced life? Which are under-represented? Is the patient spending a reasonable amount of time in activities related to work/school, family, friends, fun, her physical self (e.g., exercise), her household, her spiritual/cultural self, her intellectual self?
> 2. Which activities are highest in mastery and/or pleasure? Should the patient plan to increase the frequency of these activities?
> 3. Which activities are lowest in mastery and/or pleasure? Are these activities inherently dysphoric (e.g., ruminating in bed) and so their frequency should be reduced? Or is the patient dysphoric during potentially rewarding activities because of her automatic thoughts during those activities? In the latter case, the therapist might target the dysfunctional cognitions rather than recommending that the frequency of the activity be reduced.

In the following transcripts, the therapist reviews the completed activity chart with Sally, reinforces her conclusions of how she might better plan her time, encourages her to commit to specific changes, elicits the thoughts that might impede instituting the changes, labels her thoughts as predictions that can be tested, and gives her the choice of a follow-up homework assignment.

T: I see you filled out this activity chart every day. That's good. Did you have a chance to look it over?

P: Yeah. I realized I was spending a whole lot more time in bed than I used to.

T: And does staying in bed give you lots of pleasure and a sense of accomplishment?

P: No. The opposite. My ratings were lowest when I stayed in bed.

T: Well, that's a valuable piece of information. It seems most people who are depressed think they'll feel better if they stay in bed. But they usually find that anything is better than staying in bed. Did you learn anything else?

P: Well, I realized I used to go out a lot more with friends or just hang around a lot more with them. Now I just go from my dorm room to class to the library to the cafeteria and back to my room.

T: Does that give you an idea of what you might like to change this coming week?

P: Yeah, well, I'd like to spend more time with other people, but I just don't seem to have any energy.

T: So, you end up staying in bed?

P: Yeah.

T: Well, that's an interesting idea you have—"I don't have the energy to spend time with people." Let's write that down. Now, how could we test this idea to see if it's true?

P: I guess I could plan to spend some time with my friends and see if I could do it.

T: Would there be an advantage to doing that?

P: I might feel better.

T: Can you imagine it's later on today, and you see some friends going to class, and you think, "I could go up and ask them what they're doing tonight." What else goes through your mind?

P: They probably don't want to hang out with me.

T: Okay. Can you see how that thought might stop you from approaching them? How can you answer that thought?

P: I don't know.

T: Do you have any evidence that they won't want to hang out with you?

P: No, not really. Unless they've got other plans or too much work to do.

T: How can you find out if this idea—that they won't want to spend time with you—is right?

P: I could just go up to them and ask.

T: Okay, so if this kind of occasion comes up, you might get a chance to test two ideas. One, that you'll be too tired to spend time with friends; and two, that your friends won't want to spend time with you. Does that sound right?

P: Yes.

T: Do you want to talk specifically about when and how you'll spend more time with friends?

P: No, I can figure that out myself.

T: Okay. How about as another assignment if you try to jot down any automatic thoughts that interfere with what you've planned. Okay?

P: Okay.

T: Anything else you learned besides that you seem to be spending too much time in bed and too little time with friends?

P: I'm watching too much TV—and not enjoying it too much.

T: Anything you'd like to try to replace it with this week?

P: I really don't know.

T: I notice you don't seem to be spending much time doing physical activities—is that right?

P: Yeah. I used to run most mornings or swim.

T: What's gotten in the way of your doing these things lately?

P: Same thing as before, I guess. I've felt really tired. And I didn't think I'd enjoy it.

T: Would you like to plan more exercise then?

P: (*Nods and writes it down.*)

T: Now how likely is it that you'll make plans to see friends and do more physical activities this week?

P: Oh, I will.

T: Do you want to write them in on a blank activity chart now so you'll be more likely to commit to them?

P: No, I don't need to. I'll do them.

T: Would it be helpful this week to fill out an activity form again with accomplishment and pleasure ratings—or would you like to keep track just of those new activities we agreed on today?

P: I'll keep track of the new activities.

T: Okay. How do you want to keep track?

In this segment, the therapist leads Sally to draw conclusions from her activity monitoring. Some patients need more guidance than others to do this (e.g., "Do you notice how much time you spent in bed this week? What were your ratings like then? What change do you think you might like to try this week?"). Here the therapist guides Sally to make specific changes and plans and helps her identify automatic thoughts that might hinder her. Then he elicits her agreement to test the validity of her negative predictions and gives her a choice about monitoring activities in the coming week.

When reviewing the activity monitor, the therapist is alert for distressing automatic thoughts that might have interfered with the patient's pleasure or mastery. Had her scores been lower than he would have predicted for a given activity, the therapist would have elicited the patient's automatic thoughts during that activity.

T: I see here under "homework in library" yesterday, you gave a 1 for both pleasure and sense of accomplishment. What were you doing then?

P: Oh. I was working on a paper for economics.

T: The scores look much lower than for the other work you did this week.

P: Yeah.

T: Do you remember what was going through your mind as you were working on the paper?

P: No, not really.

T: Can you picture yourself right now, in the library? It's 1:00 yesterday; where are you sitting?

P: In the 4th-floor stacks, at a little study carrel.

T: Can you see yourself sitting there? Are you reading or staring at your paper or what?

P: I'm leaning back, staring at my papers.

T: How are you feeling?

P: Kind of disgusted.

T: And what's going through your mind?

P: I don't want to do this. It is so boring. I hate this paper. I just can't do it.

T: Okay, you've started working. It's about 1:30. What's happening now?

P: I've written like half a page. I'm thinking, "What a waste of time. This is really stupid. I can't stand this."

T: And how are you feeling?

P: Disgusted.

T: No *wonder* your scores were so low. Do you see how your thoughts affected your mood?

P: Yeah. I guess I was psyching myself up to hate what I was doing.

T: What would your mood have been like if you'd been thinking, "Hey, that's pretty good. I actually wrote half a page and I didn't think I'd be able to write anything. Now I have the start of a first draft. I've done the hardest part."

P: I probably would have felt better.

T: Okay, how about this week when you notice you're feeling down, if you tune into what's going through your head and jot down your thoughts?

P: All right.

T: Now, looking at your activity form, were there any other activities this past week where you think your thoughts might have interfered with your sense of accomplishment or pleasure?

In this portion, the therapist uses the activity chart to identify situations in which automatic thoughts have interfered with pleasure and mastery. He then uses imagery to help the patient recall the automatic thoughts and demonstrates that different thoughts would have affected the patient's mood more positively. Finally, he sets up a homework assignment for the patient to monitor her automatic thoughts and also questions whether other activities in the previous week may have been tainted by negative thoughts.

Measuring Moods Using the Activity Chart

For some patients, it is helpful to use the activity form to investigate the occurrence of a specific mood. For example, a patient with an anxiety disorder might fill in the boxes listing activities and level of anxiety 0–10. A patient who is chronically irritated or angry might do likewise, with a 0–10 anger scale. Using such a scale is particularly useful for patients who either do not seem to notice small to moderate shifts in affect or patients who chronically over- or underestimate degrees of emotion. Patients with rapidly changing moods might find it useful to list activities and the *predominant* mood they experienced for each activity.

Scheduling Activities

The same activity chart can be used to schedule activities. Instead of monitoring her activities during the week, the patient plans and writes in activities for the coming week, such as pleasurable activities (especially for depressed patients), tasks that must be done, socializing, therapy homework, exercise, or previously avoided activities. The therapist may also ask the patient if she wants to keep a parallel activity (monitoring) chart, as described previously, recording either all her activities or just the planned ones she actually did.

If the therapist considers it worthwhile, he can have the patient *predict* levels of mastery and pleasure or mood on a chart and then record *actual* ratings on another. These comparisons can be a useful source of data.

T: Let's take a look now at your predictions on the first activity chart and what actually *happened* on the second one.

P: (*Nods.*)

T: Let's see . . . it looks as if you predicted very low scores, mostly 0's to 3's, for these three times you scheduled to meet your friends. What actually did happen?

P: Actually, I had a better time than I'd thought—my pleasure scores were 3's to 5's.

T: What does that tell you?

P: I guess I'm not a good predictor. I thought I wouldn't enjoy myself, but I did, at least some.

T: Would you like to schedule more social activities for this coming week?

P: Actually, I already did. I made plans with those same friends for next week.

T: Good. Do you see what could have happened—and, in fact, what was happening before you came to therapy? You kept predicting that you'd have a lousy time with your friends so you didn't make any plans; in fact, you turned down their overtures. It sounds as if homework helped you test your ideas; you found it was wrong that you'd have a lousy time, and then you went ahead and scheduled more on your own. Is that right?

P: Yes. I'm beginning to realize that I make a lot of negative predictions. But that reminds me, I wanted to talk about one prediction which actually turned out worse.

T: Okay, when was that?

P: I predicted that I'd get 4's in accomplishment and pleasure when I went running over the weekend. But both were 1's.

T: Do you have any idea why?

P: Not really.

T: How were you feeling when you were running?

P: Mostly sad.

T: And what was going through your mind?

P: I don't know. I wasn't feeling very good. I got winded real easily. I couldn't believe how hard it was.

T: Did you have thoughts like that—"I don't feel very good," "I'm winded," "This is hard"?

P: Yeah, I think so.

T: Anything else go through your mind?

P: I remembered how easy it used to be. I could go 2 or 3 miles without getting too winded.

T: Did you have a memory, an image of how it used to be?

P: Yeah. I'm in really bad shape now. It's going to be so hard to get back in shape. I'm not sure I'll *ever* be able to get back in shape.

T: Okay, let me see if I understand. Here in my office you thought you'd get a moderate sense of accomplishment and pleasure when you went running. But, instead, you got very little. It sounds as if you were having thoughts which interfered, such as, "This is hard," "I'm real winded," "I used to do this easily," "I'm in such bad shape now," "Maybe I'll never be able to get back in shape." And these thoughts made you feel sad. Does that sound right?

P: Yeah.

In this last part, the therapist uses the activity chart as a vehicle for identifying a number of automatic thoughts that were undermining the patient's enjoyment of an activity. In the next segment, he will help her evaluate the key cognition, "Maybe I'll never be able to get back in shape." He'll also teach her to compare herself to how she was at her worst point instead of at her best point.

DISTRACTION AND REFOCUSING

As described in Chapter 8, it is usually best for the patient to evaluate her automatic thoughts on the spot and modify her thinking. In many situations, however, this strategy is unfeasible and refocusing attention, distraction, or reading coping cards is indicated.

Refocusing is particularly useful in situations in which concentration is needed for the task at hand, such as completing a work assignment, carrying on a conversation, or driving. The therapist teaches the patient to refocus on the immediate task—deliberately turning her attention to the report she is writing, to what her fellow conversationalist is saying, to the road ahead. The therapist rehearses the strategy with the patient, trying to elicit how she has refocused her attention in the past or how she believes she can do so in the future.

T: Okay, so one alternative when you're feeling anxious in class is to answer back those thoughts. But sometimes you may be better off just changing your focus to what's going on in class. Have you done this before, made an effort to concentrate on the class?

P: Ah . . . yeah, I guess so.

T: How did you do that?

P: Well, it helps if I start taking lots of notes.

T: Good. How about this week if you try *not* to let yourself just feel overwhelmed by your negative thoughts and anxiety and sadness, but instead either answer back your thoughts or refocus and take lots of notes, or both.

P: Okay.

T: How will you remember to do that?

At other times, when the patient's affect is overwhelming and there is no immediate task at hand, distraction may be useful. Again, the therapist generally elicits what has worked for the patient in the past and then offers other suggestions, if needed.

T: Okay, you did the Dysfunctional Thought Record, but you still felt pretty anxious?

P: Yeah.

T: Maybe later in this session we'll talk about why you might not feel better after doing a thought record, but for now, I'd like to talk about what else you can do to reduce your anxiety. Okay?

P: Yeah, that would help.

T: Tell me, Sally, what have you done in the past to distract yourself when you've felt bad?

P: Usually, I turn on the TV.

T: How well does that usually work?

P: Sometimes I can lose myself and feel better, sometimes not.

T: Okay, if it doesn't work well, what else do you try?

P: Sometimes I pick up the newspaper or do a crossword puzzle, but that doesn't always work either.

T: Any other ideas?

P: . . . No, not really.

T: Let me mention some things that other people find helpful. You might try one or two of these things as an experiment this week: take a walk or go running, call a friend on the phone, clean your closet or desk or rearrange shelves, balance your checkbook, go to the grocery store, knock on a neighbor's door. What do you think? Do you want to try any of these things this week?

P: Yeah. I think running might help. I used to do that.

The better solution for dysphoria is not merely to push thoughts out of mind by refocusing or distraction. Patients need a variety of tools to reduce their dysphoria, particularly when cognitive restructuring is impractical or ineffective. One caveat, however, is that some patients do tend to rely too heavily on these alternative techniques to alleviate their distress, rather than evaluating and modifying their automatic thoughts. A brief discussion such as the following usually helps:

T: So, what you're saying is that you tend to try to push your thoughts out of your mind when you're feeling sad. Is that right?

P: Yes.

T: And do these thoughts, for example, that you can't do something, vanish from your mind completely?

P: No, they usually come back.

T: So, you're not really pushing them completely out of mind, just to the back of your mind, where they wait for another opportunity to pop out and make you miserable?

P: I guess so.

T: I wonder this week if you would be willing, at least some of the time, to stop distracting yourself and instead really work on these thoughts, evaluate them as you've been learning to do in session?

P: Okay.

T: Even if it's impossible to do a Dysfunctional Thought Record at the time, maybe you could do it as soon as you have a free moment.

RELAXATION

Many patients benefit from learning relaxation techniques, described in detail elsewhere (Benson, 1975; Jacobson, 1974). As with all the techniques described in this volume, relaxation exercises should be taught and practiced in session, where problems can be dealt with and efficacy can be assessed.

The therapist should also be aware that some patients experience a paradoxical arousal effect from relaxation exercises; they actually become more tense and anxious (Clark, 1989). As with all techniques, the therapist proposes that the patient try relaxation as an experiment; either it will help reduce anxiety or it will lead to anxious thoughts which can be evaluated.

COPING CARDS

Coping cards are usually 3" × 5" notecards which a patient keeps nearby (often in a desk drawer, pocket, or purse or posted on a bathroom mirror, refrigerator, or car dashboard). She is encouraged to read them on both a regular basis (e.g., three times a day) and as needed. These cards can take several forms, three of which are described here: writing a key automatic thought or belief on one side with its adaptive response on the other, devising behavioral strategies to use in a specific problematic situation, and composing self-instructions to activate the patient.

Coping Card 1: Automatic Thought–Adaptive Response

When a patient cannot evaluate distressing thoughts and when distraction or refocusing is not preferable, the patient can read a coping card (see Figures 12.4 and 12.5) that she and the therapist have composed in advance. It is desirable for the patient to read the card on a regular basis as well so she will be more likely to integrate it into her thinking.

T: Do you think it would be helpful to have a card to read to remind yourself how to respond to this thought, "I can't do this," when you're reading your economics textbook?

P: Yeah.

T: Okay, how about if you take this card and write, "I can't do this," on one side.

P: (*Does so.*)

T: Now, what did we just discuss that would be good for you to remember?

Following the discussion, the patient summarizes the most important points to put on the reverse side of the card. Then the therapist and patient discuss when it would be helpful to read the card, for example, at breakfast, lunch, dinner, and at strategic points during the day: before she gathers her books to go to the library, when she first sits down, and when she gets to a part of the text that is difficult.

COPING CARD 1

(Side 1) **Automatic thought** *I can't do this.*

(Side 2) **Adaptive response** *Well, I might feel like I can't do it, but it may not be true. Lots of times in the past I've thought I couldn't read and understand this text, but if I actually go ahead and open the book and start to read, I do understand it, at least to some extent. It may be difficult, but it's probably not true that I can't do it at all. The worst that'll happen is I'll start to read and not understand it, but then I can either stop or ask someone about it or do some other work instead. That would be better than not trying it at all. Negative thinking just undermines my motivation. I should go ahead and test the idea I can't do it.*

FIGURE 12.4. Coping card 1.

Coping Card 2: Coping Strategies

A second type of coping card lists techniques for a patient to try when she is in a difficult situation (Figure 12.5). In a collaborative manner, the therapist and patient develop such a card so the patient can remember strategies that were discussed in session. The therapist asks the patient what she thinks she can do in a particular situation and then adds suggestions. The patient writes the coping card, using the ideas she thinks will be useful.

T: We've just talked about a number of things you can do when you're feeling very anxious. Would it help you to write them on a card which you could pull out as a reminder?

P: Yeah.

T: Here's a card. How about writing at the top, "Strategies for when I'm anxious." Now what would you like to write under it?

Coping Card 3: Instructions to Activate a Patient

When a patient is feeling unmotivated, a coping card can help her get activated (Figure 12.5). Again, this card is developed collaboratively. ("Sally, do you think it would help to write on a card the things we've just

COPING CARD 2

Strategies for when I'm anxious

1. Do a Dysfunctional Thought Record.
2. Read coping cards.
3. Call [friend].
4. Go for a walk or run.

COPING CARD 3

When I want to ask the professor for help

1. Remind myself it's no big deal. The worst that'll happen is he'll act gruff.
2. Remember, this is an experiment. Even if it doesn't work this time, it's good practice for me.
3. If he is gruff, it probably has nothing to do with me. He may be busy or irritated by something else.
4. Even if he won't help me, so what? It's his failure as a professor, not mine as a student. It means he isn't doing his job properly.
5. So I should go knock on his door now. Remember, at worst, it's good practice.

FIGURE 12.5. Coping cards 2 and 3.

discussed about going to your professor?") The therapist may have to spend some time motivating the patient to read the card itself, by examining advantages and disadvantages of reading the card, specifying when she should read it, and eliciting and responding to predicted automatic thoughts that may inhibit her use of the card.

GRADED EXPOSURE

In order to reach a goal, it is usually necessary to accomplish a number of steps along the way. Patients tend to become overwhelmed when they focus on how far they are from a goal instead of focusing on their current step. A graphic depiction of the steps is often reassuring to the patient (see Figure 12.6).

T: Sally, it sounds like it's pretty scary just thinking about voluntarily talking in class, though it's something you want to be able to do.

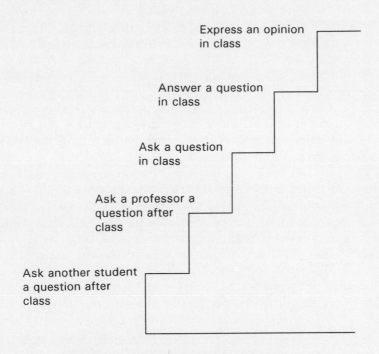

FIGURE 12.6. Breaking down goals into steps.

P: Yeah.

T: I wonder how we could break it down into steps; for example, could you start by just asking a question *after* class, either to another student or to the professor?

P: Yeah. I guess I could do that.

T: What could the next step be? [The therapist guides Sally in identifying the steps presented in Figure 12.6.]

T: Does it still seem scary to think about talking in class?

P: Yeah, some.

T: (*Draws a staircase.*) Okay, here's what you have to remember. You're going to start down here, doing something that's just a little hard, and you'll get really comfortable on this step before trying the next step, and so on. And remember, before you try the final step, you'll have gotten really good at the step just below it. Okay?

P: Uh huh.

T: So every time you start thinking about the final goal, how about reminding yourself of this staircase and especially of the step you're now on and how you're going to go up the staircase one step at a time. Do you think that'll help bring down the anxiety?

The therapist generally suggests starting with an activity that is associated with low to moderate anxiety, practicing this step every day or even several times a day until the patient's anxiety has decreased significantly. The patient then attempts the next task in the hierarchy until she can do it with relative ease.

Therapist and patient may discuss various coping techniques to use before, during, and after each task: Dysfunctional Thought Records, coping cards, relaxation exercises, etc. For particularly avoidant patients, covert rehearsal (Chapter 14) to identify either dysphoric automatic thoughts or excuses not to do an assignment is useful. In addition, the therapist may find that the patient is more likely to do daily work on a graded exposure hierarchy if she is asked to fill out an activity chart. A blank activity chart may be used or a custom-made monitor can be quickly drawn. The monitor can be simple, listing just the date, activity, and level of anxiety, or it can be more elaborate (see Figure 12.7). In a more elaborate monitor, the patient can also be instructed to record and then cross off predictions that did not come true, a task that further reminds the patient of the inaccuracy of many of her thoughts. Detailed descriptions of the process used to develop agoraphobic hierarchies can be found in various sources (e.g., Goldstein & Stainback, 1987).

ROLE-PLAYING

Role-playing is a technique that can be used for a wide variety of purposes. Descriptions of role-playing can be found throughout this volume, including role-playing to uncover automatic thoughts, to develop a rational response, and to modify intermediate and core beliefs. Role-playing is also useful in learning and practicing social skills.

Some patients have weak social skills in general, or are proficient at one style of communication but lack skills to adapt their style when needed. Sally, for example, is quite skilled in normal social conversation and situations that call for a caring, empathic stance. She is far less skilled, however, in situations in which assertion is appropriate. The therapist and she practice a number of role-plays to practice assertiveness, as this skill is one of her therapy goals.

Date	Activity	Predicted level of anxiety 0–100	Actual level of anxiety 1–100	Predictions	Coping techniques used
4/4	Asking questions in class	80	50	I won't be able to do it. Nothing will come out of my mouth. I'll make a fool of myself.	DTR before class. Read coping cards before class.

FIGURE 12.7. Custom-made monitor.

P: I don't even know how I'd begin to talk to my professor.

T: Well, you want him to help you understand this concept better, right? What could you say?

P: . . . I don't know.

T: Well, how about if we do a role-play. I'll be you; you play your professor. You can play him as being as unreasonable as you'd like.

P: Okay.

T: I'll start: Uh, Professor X, could you explain this concept?

P: (*Gruffly.*) I did that already last week in class. Weren't you there?

T: Actually, I was. But, I don't understand it well enough yet.

P: Well, you should go read the chapter in your textbook.

T: I've done that already. It didn't help enough either. That's why I'm here now.

P: Okay, what don't you understand about it?

T: I tried to think of a specific question before I came, but I couldn't quite think of how to phrase it. Could you spend a couple of minutes just describing it, and then I can see if I can put it in my own words?

P: You know, I don't have much time now. Why don't you see someone else in the class?

T: I'd rather get it straight from you. That's why I came now during office hours. But, if you'd rather, I could come back on Thursday when you have office hours again.

P: This is a simple concept. You should really ask some other student.

T: I'll try that first. If I need more help, I'll come back Thursday. . . . . Okay, out of role. Let's review what I did and then we can switch roles.

Before teaching a patient social skills, the therapist assesses the level of skill the patient already has. Many patients know precisely what to do and say but have difficulty using this knowledge because of dysfunctional assumptions (e.g., "If I express an opinion, I'll get shot down"; "If I assert myself, the other person will be hurt/get mad/think I'm out of line"). One way of assessing skills is to have the patient assume a positive outcome: "If you knew for sure the teaching assistant would be glad to talk to you, what would you say?" "If you really believed it was your right to get help, what would you say?" "If you knew the professor would back down and realize he was being unreasonable, what would you say?"

Another indication that the problem is associated with dysfunctional beliefs rather than with a skill deficit is the patient's use of these skills in another context. A patient may be quite appropriately assertive at work, for example, but not with friends. In this case, the therapist might not need to use role-playing to teach assertiveness skills (though he could use role-playing to have the patient identify her automatic thoughts while she is being assertive or to predict thoughts and feelings of the other person when roles are switched).

USING THE "PIE" TECHNIQUE

It is often helpful to patients to see their ideas in graphic form. A pie chart can be used in many ways, for instance, in helping the patient set goals or in determining relative responsibility for a given outcome, both of which are illustrated below. (See Figure 12.8.)

Setting Goals

When a patient has difficulty specifying her problems and what changes she would like to make in her life, or when she lacks insight into how imbalanced her life is, she may benefit from a graphic depiction of her ideal versus actual expenditure of time.

T: Sally, it sounds as if you know your life isn't quite in balance, but you don't know what to change.

P: Right.

T: How about if we draw a pie diagram to help figure it out?

P: Okay.

T: First, we'll create a diagram of your life now, then an ideal one. Think about how much time you are actually spending in these areas:

Work/school	Taking care of your physical
Friends	self
Fun	Taking care of your household
Family	Taking care of your spiritual/
Other interests	cultural/intellectual side

T: Can you draw a pie and put in divisions to give me a *rough* idea of how you're spending your time now? (*Does so.*)

T: Okay, next, what would you change about it in an ideal world?

P: Well . . . I guess I'd work less, probably try to have more fun . . . spend more time with friends, exercise more, spend more time volunteering at the elementary school—

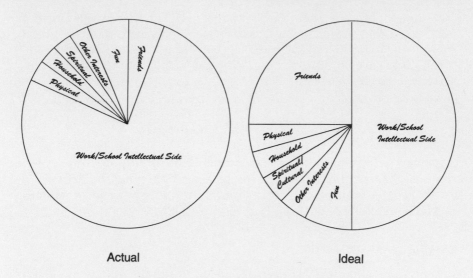

Actual   Ideal

FIGURE 12.8. Use of pie chart in setting goals.

T: Good. How would that look on this ideal pie?

P: (*Fills in "Ideal Pie."*) But I'm afraid if I spend less time working, I'll do even worse at school.

T: Okay, let's write down that prediction. Now, you may be right, in which case you could always go back to the amount of studying you're doing now. Or, you may be wrong. It's possible if you work less and do more pleasurable things, that your mood will improve. If your mood improves, is it possible that you might concentrate better and study more efficiently? What do you think?

P: I'm not sure.

T: In any case, we can test your prediction and see what happens.

P: I know for a fact that I'm not studying too efficiently right now.

T: Then it may well be that once we get your life back in balance and you're getting positive inputs from doing things you like, that you'll be able to do better with less work. [The therapist and patient now set specific goals to move patient's expenditure of time closer to her ideal.]

Examining the Contribution of Various Factors to a Negative Outcome

Another pie technique allows the patient to see graphically the possible causes for a given outcome (see Figure 12.9).

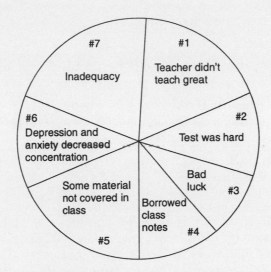

FIGURE 12.9. Pie chart for causality.

T: Sally, how much do you believe you got a C on your exam because you're basically inadequate?

P: Oh, close to 100%.

T: I wonder if there might be any other reasons?

P: . . . Well, there were some things on it that we had never really covered in class.

T: Okay, anything else?

P: I missed two classes, so I had to borrow notes and Lisa's notes weren't that good.

T: Anything else?

P: I don't know. I studied some things a lot that turned out not to be on the exam.

T: Sounds like you weren't very lucky in that regard.

P: No, and I only studied a little things that were on the exam. I guessed wrong.

T: Any other reason to explain why you didn't do as well as you would have liked?

P: Hmmm. Can't think of any.

T: Did everyone else do pretty well?

P: I don't know.

T: Would you say it was a hard test?

P: Yeah, too hard.

T: Would you say the professor had done a really good job of explaining the material?

P: No. I don't think he did a great job. I had to rely on the readings, mostly. A couple of times, I heard people saying that they hadn't been able to follow what he was talking about.

T: I wonder if you also might have trouble concentrating because of your depression and anxiety?

P: Definitely.

T: Okay, let's see how all this would look graphically. Here's a pie; let's have you divide up sections to explain why you got a C on the exam, including (1) the professor didn't teach that great; (2) the test was really hard; (3) you had bad luck because you happened not to study as much the material that turned out to be on the exam; (4) you borrowed class notes that weren't great; (5) there was material on the exam that wasn't even covered in class; (6) your depression and anxiety interfered with your concentration; and (7) at heart, you're an inadequate person. (*The patient fills in pie diagram, Figure 12.9.*)

T: Looks like you divided up the sections pretty evenly. How much do you believe now that you got a C on the exam because you're an inadequate person?

P: Less. 50%, maybe.

T: Good. That's quite a drop.

When investigating the contribution of alternative explanations, the therapist has the patient estimate the dysfunctional attribution (in this case, "I'm inadequate") last so she will more fully consider all explanations.

FUNCTIONAL COMPARISONS OF THE SELF AND POSITIVE SELF-STATEMENT LOGS

Patients with psychiatric disorders have a negative bias in information processing, especially when evaluating themselves. They tend to notice data that could be construed as negative and to ignore or discount or even forget information that is positive. In addition, they often make one of two dysfunctional comparisons: They compare themselves at present with how they were before the onset of their disorder or they compare themselves with others who do not have a psychiatric disorder. This negative attentional bias helps to maintain or increase their dysphoria.

Changing the Self-Comparison

In the following transcript, the therapist helps the patient see that her selective negative attention and comparisons are dysfunctional. He then teaches her to make more functional comparisons (with herself at her worst point) and to keep a positive self-statement log.

T: Sally, it sounds as if you're pretty down on yourself. Do you think there's anything you did this week that you deserve credit for?

P: Well, I did finish my lit paper.

T: Anything else?

P: Ummm . . . Can't think of anything.

T: I wonder if you might not have noticed some things.

P: I don't know.

T: For instance, how many classes did you go to?

P: All of them.

T: In how many did you take notes?

P: All of them.

T: Was that easy to do? Or did you have to push yourself to go and concentrate?

P: It was hard. But I should have been able to do it easily. No one else probably had to push.

T: Oh. . . . Sounds as if you might be comparing yourself with other people again. Do you do that a lot?

P: Yeah, I guess so.

T: Does that seem like a fair comparison to you? Would you be as hard on yourself, for example, if you had to push yourself to go to class and concentrate if you had pneumonia?

P: No, I'd have a legitimate reason to be tired.

T: Exactly. I wonder if you have a legitimate reason to be tired now? Maybe you *do* deserve credit when you push yourself. Do you remember at the first session when we talked about the symptoms of depression: tiredness, low energy, trouble concentrating, disturbances in sleep and appetite, and so on?

P: Uh huh.

T: So maybe you *do* deserve credit for pushing ahead given that you are depressed?

P: I hadn't thought of it that way.

T: Okay, let's go over two things now: what to do when you compare yourself with others and how to keep track of what you deserve credit for. Okay, what happens to your mood when you compare yourself to others, for example, when you think, "No one else has to push herself to go to class and take notes?"

P: I feel pretty bad.

T: And what would happen if you said to yourself, "Now wait a minute. That's not a reasonable comparison. Let me compare myself to *me* at my worst point, when I was staying in bed all day and missing a lot of classes."

P: Well, I'd realize that I'm doing more now.

T: And would your mood get worse?

P: No, probably better.

T: Would you like to try this comparison for homework?

P: Uh huh.

T: Okay, let's have you write this down on your assignment sheet, "Catch myself comparing me to other nondepressed people. Then remind myself this isn't reasonable and compare myself to me at my worst point instead."

The patient may also have automatic thoughts in which she compares herself at present to where she would like to be (e.g., "I should be able to read this chapter easily"), or to where she was before she got depressed (e.g., "This used to be so easy for me"). Again, the therapist focuses her attention on how far she has progressed since her worst point rather than on how far she is from her best point or on how far she has to go.

Part of the previous transcript was predicated on the therapist's knowledge that Sally had already improved somewhat. In another situation, the therapist ascertains when the worst point was: "When was the worst point for you? What was your life like then?" "What were you doing/not doing then?" If the patient accurately replies that the worst point ever was right now, the therapist modifies his approach: "It sounds as if you feel pretty down when you compare yourself with other people or with how you wish you were. I wonder if it might be helpful at these times to remind yourself that you have a goal list and that together we're developing a plan to help you make some changes. If you reminded

yourself that you and I are a team working to get you to where you want
to be, what could happen to your mood?"

Positive Self-Statement Logs

Positive self-statement logs are simply daily lists of positive things the
patient is doing or items she deserves credit for. (See Figure 12.10.) As
with all assignments, the therapist first explains the rationale:

T: Sally, I'd like to describe a homework assignment that I think could
help. You know, we've talked about how really good you are at
criticizing yourself and finding fault. Now, what happens to your mood
every time you have a thought like, "I should be doing this better," or
"I did a lousy job on that"?

P: I feel worse.

T: Right. And what would happen, do you think, if you started noticing
more good things you're doing?

P: I'd probably feel better.

T: Okay, now would you say that it would be reasonable for *me* to give
myself credit if I were tired from either pneumonia or depression, but
I pushed ahead anyway and got out of bed and came to work and saw
my patients and wrote letters and so on?

P: Sure.

T: Even if I didn't do these things as well as usual?

P: Well, sure.

T: Because I suppose I could have stayed in bed and pulled the covers
over my head instead.

P: Right.

CREDIT LIST

(Things that I did that were positive or were a little hard but I did them anyway)

1. Tried to follow what was said in statistics class.
2. Finished typing paper and handed it in.
3. Talked to Julia at lunch.
4. Called Jon to confirm chemistry assignment.
5. Cooked dinner instead of taking a nap.
6. Read Chapter 5 of econ book.

FIGURE 12.10. Sally's credit list.

T: Now, does that same thing apply to you? Do *you* deserve credit for pushing ahead?

P: I guess so.

T: You know, it's probably hard for you to remember to give yourself credit outside of our session. That's why I'm suggesting you keep a written list of things you deserve credit for. What do you think?

P: I could try it.

T: Here, let's try it now, if that's okay with you. What do you want to call it—Credit List? Positive Self-Statement Log? Something else?

P: Oh, Credit List, I guess.

T: Good. Now on this list you can either just write positive things you've done or you can think to yourself, "What did I do today that was even a little hard, but I did it anyway?"

P: Okay. (*Writes instructions down.*)

T: Let's start with today. What have you already done today?

P: (*Writes as she speaks.*) Let's see, I went to my statistics class . . . it was kind of hard to follow, but I tried. . . . I finished typing my paper and handed it in. . . . I talked to my roommate's friend who had lunch with us—

T: That's a good start. How do you feel about doing this every day?

P: Okay.

T: I think that you'll remember things ten times better if you write them down immediately. But if you can't, you might at least try to write things down at lunch, dinner, and before bed. Think you can do that?

P: Yeah.

T: Think you need to write down *why* you're doing this assignment?

P: No, I'll remember. It makes me focus on good things and that makes me feel better.

Completing positive self-statement logs early in therapy also helps prepare patients for the later task of uncovering positive data for the Core Belief Worksheet (Chapter 11).

In summary, there are many cognitive and behavioral techniques; this volume describes the most common. Readers are encouraged to do additional reading to add to their repertoire.

Chapter 13

IMAGERY

M any patients experience automatic thoughts not only as unspoken words in their mind but also in the form of mental pictures or images (Beck & Emery, 1985). Sally had the thought, "My professor will think I'm imposing on him if I ask for help." Upon questioning, her therapist determined that Sally, along with these verbal automatic thoughts, had simultaneously envisioned her professor standing tall over her, scowling, and looking quite annoyed as she asked a question. This image was an imaginal automatic thought.

This chapter demonstrates how to teach patients to identify their spontaneous images and how to intervene therapeutically with both spontaneous and induced images. Although many patients have visual images, few report them. Merely asking about images, even repeatedly, sometimes is not sufficient to elicit them. Images usually are quite brief and are often upsetting; many patients push them out of mind quite quickly. Failure to identify and respond to upsetting images may result in continued distress for the patient. The therapist begins to educate the patient about images in the first session (see Chapter 3).

IDENTIFYING IMAGES

In order to teach patients how to recognize and intervene with their distressing images, the therapist tries either to elicit a spontaneous image a patient has had or to induce an image in session. In the following transcript, the therapist seeks to discover whether Sally has had a spontaneous image simultaneous with a verbal automatic thought.

THERAPIST: So you had the thought, "He'll think I'm imposing on him if I ask for help," and you felt anxious?

PATIENT: Yes.

T: I wonder, when you had that thought, did you get a picture in your head?

P: I'm not sure what you mean.

T: Did you imagine what your professor might look like when you asked him for help? Did he look happy? (*Providing a possibility opposite to the expected one to help the patient focus.*)

P: No, he was scowling.

T: Did you imagine anything else? Where, for example, did you picture this taking place, in the classroom?

P: No. I pictured myself knocking on the door of his office and going in and telling him I didn't understand something he had talked about in class.

T: And then what?

P: Well, I saw him standing over me, real tall, and scowling down at me.

T: Anything else?

P: No, that's all.

T: Okay. That picture, or imagining, is what we call an image.

At times, patients fail to grasp the concept when the therapist only uses the word "image." Synonyms include mental picture, daydream, fantasy, imagining, and memory. Had Sally failed to report an image, her therapist might have tried using one of these different words. Or he might have chosen to induce an image (if a therapeutic goal for that session was to help her recognize images). He could have induced a neutral or positive image ("Describe for me what the outside of your home looks like," or "Imagine you're walking into this building. What do you see?"). Or, the therapist might have tried to induce an image about a distressing situation as below:

T: Did you imagine what your professor might look like when you asked him for help? Did he look happy?

P: I don't think I pictured what he looked like.

T: Could you picture it now? Can you imagine going up to him? When would you approach him, anyway? (*Helping the patient to think very specifically.*)

P: Oh, probably on Tuesday. That's when he has office hours.

T: So he'd be in his office?

P: Yeah.

T: What building is he in?

P: Bennett Hall.

T: Okay, can you picture it now? It's Tuesday, you're coming up to Bennett Hall. . . . You're coming to his office. . . . Can you see it in your mind? Is the door open or closed?

P: Closed.

T: Okay, can you see yourself knocking on the door? What does he say when he hears your knock?

P: He says, "Come in." (*Imitates professor's gruff voice.*)

T: Okay, can you see yourself go in? What does his face look like?

P: He's scowling.

T: And then what happens? [The therapist and patient follow the image out to its most distressing point.] Okay, this scene you've just visualized is what we call an image. Do you think you might have had an image like this when you were considering going to see him this week?

P: Maybe . . . I'm not sure.

T: How about for homework if you look for images when you realize you're getting upset, along with looking for automatic thoughts.

P: Okay.

EDUCATING PATIENTS ABOUT IMAGERY

Some patients can identify images but do not report them to therapists because their images are graphic and distressing. They may be reluctant to reexperience the distress or fear the therapist will view them as disturbed. If the therapist suspects either scenario, he normalizes the experience of images.

T: Sally, I don't know whether or not you *are* having images. Most people do but usually they're more aware of the emotion that accompanies the image than they are of the image itself. Sometimes, images seem pretty strange, but actually it's common to have all kinds of images— sad, scary, even violent ones. The only problem is if you think *you're* strange for having the images. Can you recall any images you've had recently?

P: No, I don't think so.

T: Well, we've agreed this week that you're going to be on the lookout for images when you notice your mood changing. If you *are* having distressing images, I'll teach you what you can do about them.

Normalizing and teaching the patient about images help to reduce her anxiety and make it more likely that she will be able to identify the images. In the previous transcript, the therapist indicates that the patient will learn to respond to images, implying that she can gain control over her distress.

The therapist must often be diligent in teaching patients to identify images until they "catch on." Most patients simply are unaware of images initially, and many therapists, after a few tries, abandon the attempt. If the therapist himself gets a visual image as the patient is describing a situation, he can use his images as a cue to probe further for an image the patient may have experienced.

T: Sally, as you were just describing how you're afraid your roommate will react, I got a picture of her in *my* head, even though I don't know her. Have you been imagining how she might look when you bring up the problem of noise with her?

If the patient continues to have difficulty identifying spontaneous images, the therapist might induce an image around a less threatening situation. "Did you imagine what I might look like even before you met me? Or, what this office might look like? . . . Describe this picture to me. . . . This picture is what we call an image." An alternative is to have the patient recall a recent event: "How did you get here today? Can you see yourself getting on the bus? How crowded was it? In what part of the bus did you sit? What did the closest person to you look like? Can you get a picture of this?"

RESPONDING TO SPONTANEOUS IMAGES

Once the therapist has ascertained that a patient has frequent, distressing images, he teaches her several ways of responding to them, using a rationale similar to the following:

T: Sally, I'd like to go over with you different things you can do when you notice a distressing image. It's hard to know in advance for any given image which technique will be the most helpful, so in the next couple of sessions, we'll try a few. Okay?

There are several techniques patients can learn to respond to their spontaneous images. The first six techniques help patients reduce their distress by viewing a situation in a different way; the last one offers temporary respite by having the patient focus on something else. The therapist also advises the patient that she will need to practice the techniques many times in and out of session in order for her to use them effectively.

Following Images to Completion

This technique is often the most helpful one and therefore may be taught first. It can help the therapist and patient conceptualize the patient's problem better, lead to cognitive restructuring of the image, and provide relief. The therapist encourages the patient to continue imagining a spontaneous image until one of two things occurs: Either the patient imagines getting through a crisis and feels better or she imagines an ultimate catastrophe, such as death. (If the latter happens, the therapist can then explore the feared consequences and meaning of the ultimate catastrophe and intervene further.) The first transcript illustrates the first scenario; the patient imagines getting through a particular difficulty.

T: Okay, Sally, can you get that image in mind again? Tell it to me aloud as you imagine it as vividly as possible.

P: I'm sitting in class. My professor is passing out the exam. I'm looking at it. My mind is going blank. I read the first question. Nothing is making sense. I see everyone else busy writing. I'm thinking, "I'm paralyzed. I'm going to fail."

T: And you're feeling . . . ?

P: Really, really anxious.

T: Anything else happen?

P: No.

T: Okay. This is very typical. You've stopped the image at the very *worst* point, where you're feeling blank and paralyzed. Now what I want you to do is imagine what happens next.

P: Hmmm. I'm not sure.

T: Well, do you stay that way for the whole hour?

P: No, I guess not.

T: Can you picture what happens next? . . . If you're looking around and seeing the other students, are you actually paralyzed?

P: No, I guess not.

T: What do you see happening next?

P: I look at my exam again, but I can't focus.

T: Then what happens?

P: I blink. The first question doesn't make any sense to me.

T: Okay, then what?

P: I skip to the next question. I'm not sure of the answer.

T: Then what?

P: I keep going until I find a question I know something about.

T: Then what?

P: I guess I write the answer.

T: Can you see yourself writing the answer?

P: Yes.

T: Good. Then what?

P: I keep going until I find something else I can answer.

T: Then what?

P: I go back to the first few questions, try to write something.

T: Good. Then what?

P: Well, eventually I finish as much as I can.

T: Then what?

P: I hand in the paper.

T: And then?

P: I guess I go on to my next class.

T: And then?

P: I sit down, get out the right notebook.

T: And how are you feeling in the image now?

P: A little shaky still. I don't know how I did on the exam.

T: Better than at the start when you were feeling blank and paralyzed?

P: Oh, yeah. Much better.

T: Good. Let's review what you did. First, you recognized a distressing image which you stopped at the absolute worst point. Then you kept imagining what would happen next until you got to the point where you were feeling somewhat better. This is what we call "following the image to completion." Do you think it would help to practice this technique?

In the previous example, the patient is easily able to identify a reasonable outcome. In some cases, the therapist needs to suggest a modification of the scene:

T: Can you picture what happens next? . . . If you're looking around and seeing the other students, are you actually paralyzed?

P: I don't know. I *feel* paralyzed.

T: What do you see happening next?

P: I don't know. I just keep sitting there, feeling paralyzed.

T: Can you see yourself move around a little in the chair, take a breath, look out the window?

P: Uh huh.

T: Can you see yourself rubbing the back of your neck, making yourself less stiff?

P: Yeah.

T: Okay, are you ready now in the image to read through the test until something seems familiar?

P: Yes.

T: Are you picturing that? What happens next?

P: I find an easier question.

T: Then what?

Here the therapist introduces a new element into the image to help the patient get "unstuck." He continues in this vein until the patient can continue on her own.

As mentioned above, sometimes the patient imagines a scene that worsens, often catastrophically. The therapist then conceptualizes the meaning of the catastrophe and intervenes accordingly. This situation is exemplified by a different patient, Marie.

T: Okay, Marie, so you see yourself in the car and it's starting to drift toward the guard rail of the bridge. Now, get as clear a picture in your mind as you can. Then what happens?

P: It's getting closer. It crashes through. (*Cries softly.*)

T: (*Gently.*) Then what?

P: (*Crying.*) The car is totally wrecked.

T: (*Softly.*) And you?

P: (*Crying.*) I'm dead.

T: Then what happens?

P: I don't know. I can't see past that. (*Still crying.*)

T: Marie, I think it'll help if we try to go a little further. What's the worst part about dying in this crash?

P: My kids. They won't have a mother any more. They'll be just devastated. (*Crying harder.*)

T: (*Waits a moment.*) Do you have an image of them?

In this example, following the image to completion leads to a catastrophe. The therapist keeps gently questioning so he can determine the special significance of the catastrophe. A later example in this chapter, inducing images to provide distance, illustrates one way to deal with this type of problem. In this case, the patient reveals that she has had a new image, of her children at her funeral, feeling utterly devastated. Once again, the patient has cut off an image at the worst point. (See pp. 246–247 for an illustration of how the therapist will have the patient imagine her children [doing better] many years in the future.)

In summary, two outcomes are possible when following an image to completion. In one instance, the problem is eventually resolved and the patient feels relief. In the second instance, the problem worsens to a catastrophe, at which point the therapist seeks to discover its special significance, thus uncovering a new problem. Therapist and patient can then induce a coping image, described later in this chapter.

Jumping Ahead in Time

At times, following an image to completion is ineffective because the patient keeps imagining more and more obstacles or distressing events with no end in sight. At this point, the therapist might suggest that the patient imagine herself at some time in the near future.

T: (*Summarizing.*) Okay, Sally, when you imagine getting started on this paper, you keep seeing how hard it is and how much effort it's taking and how many problems you're having with it. Realistically, do you think you'll eventually finish the paper?

P: Yeah, probably. I might have to work day and night for a long time, though.

T: How about if you jump ahead in time and imagine finishing it. Can you picture that? What does that look like?

P: Well, I guess I see myself making the last correction. Then I go hand it in.

T: Wait a moment. Can you slow it down a little, really imagine the details, like stapling the pages or making a photocopy?

P: Okay. I'm using a computer at the Student Center so I print out two copies. I staple each one. I put the one to hand in in a manila folder. I put it in my bookbag, then put on my coat, then walk over to College Hall to hand it in.

T: Can you see yourself walking over, handing it in?

P: Yeah.

T: How do you feel in the image now?

P: Relieved . . . like a weight has been taken off my chest. A lot lighter.

T: Okay, let's review what we did. You had an image of yourself starting to work on this paper and the more you imagined, the more problems you saw and the more anxious you were getting. Then you jumped ahead in time and saw yourself finishing it, which made you feel better. How about if we have you write something down about this technique— jumping ahead in time—so you'll be able to practice it at home, too?

Coping in the Image

Another technique is to guide the patient in imagining that she is coping with the difficult situation she has spontaneously envisioned.

T: (*Summarizing.*) So you had an image of walking into the [elementary] school library with the student you've volunteered to tutor, and you're feeling at a complete loss? And then the kid acts up and starts making noise, and you feel as if he's out of control?

P: Yeah.

T: So once again, you've had an image and left yourself at the worst point?

P: Yeah, I guess I did.

T: Can we go through this image again, and this time, see if you can imagine coping with each problem as it arises.

P: Well, first the kid bangs open the library door. I guess I tell him, "Shh. There's another class in here."

T: And then what?

P: He starts veering over to the books.

T: So you—

P: I guess I take his hand and guide him to a table.

The dialogue continues in this way until the patient has successfully coped in the image. If necessary, the therapist helps by asking leading questions (as on pp. 233–234). If applicable, the therapist can guide the patient to imagine herself using tools she learned in therapy, for example, reading a coping card, using controlled breathing, and saying aloud self-instructions.

Changing the Image

Another technique involves teaching the patient to identify an image, then reimagine it, changing the ending. Doing so usually alleviates her distress. The first example is a realistic change, the second, a more "magical" change.

T: Sally, last week we talked about a couple of things you can do when you notice a distressing image. Do you remember? . . . Did you try any imagery techniques this week? . . . Let me tell you about another one—*changing the image* in some way. Can you remember any other times this week when you had a distressing image?

P: (*Pauses.*) Yeah. This morning. I was thinking about spring vacation. I can't go home. I'll have to stay here.

T: What was happening in the image?

P: I was imagining myself just sitting at my desk, alone in my room, kind of slumped over, feeling really down.

T: Anything else?

P: No, just that it's really quiet. The dorm is deserted.

T: And the image makes you feel—

P: Sad. Real sad.

T: Sally, you don't have to be at the mercy of this image. You can change it, if you want. It's as if you're a movie director: You can decide how you want it to be instead. You can change it in a magical way . . . something that couldn't really happen. Or, you can change it to a realistic image. I think if you try it, you'll feel less distressed.

P: I'm not sure I understand how.

T: Well, okay, you're sitting at your desk. What do you *wish* would happen next?

P: That my best friend calls me . . . or it turns out there are more people in the dorm and someone comes knocking on my door, and we go to dinner together.

T: Any other scenario?

P: Maybe that I remember there's some event on campus, like a softball game, and I go watch or play.

T: Those *are* much better endings. How do you think you'd feel if you imagined those things happening?

P: Better. But how do I know they'll come true?

T: Well, first of all, neither of us really knows if sitting at your desk, crying, will come true or not. What we *do* know is that *imagining* that makes you feel really sad now. Second of all, maybe we could talk now about how to make it more likely that there really *is* a better ending. What could you do so your friend might call, or a dorm mate might knock on your door, or you might go to a campus event?

Changing the image in this case leads to a productive discussion involving problem-solving.

Some images lend themselves to change that is more "magical" in nature. Altering the image in this way also usually leads to a reduction in distress and allows the patient to behave in a more productive way. An example follows:

T: (*Summarizing, using the patient's own words.*) So you have an image of your professor standing very tall over you, scowling, speaking harshly, stomping his foot, being overbearing, and the image makes you very anxious.

P: Yes.

T: Would you like to change the image? Imagine him in a different way?

P: How?

T: I don't know. . . . He kind of reminds me of a 3-year-old, having a tantrum. Can you imagine that he shrinks down in size but still is scowling, still stomping his foot?

P: (*Smiles.*) Yes.

T: Describe him to me, in detail. [Patient does so.] And how do you feel now? As anxious?

P: No, less.

T: Has it come down enough to let you go make an appointment with him?

P: Yes, I think so.

T: Okay, let's review what we just did. We started with an image you had of your professor. It sounded as if this image was so distressing that it stopped you from doing what you need to do—making an appointment with him. Then you took control of the image by changing it and your anxiety came down, enough for you to go and meet with him. We call this technique "changing the image."

Reality-Testing the Image

Here the therapist teaches the patient to treat the image like a verbal automatic thought, using standard Socratic questioning.

T: So you had an image of me frowning and looking disapproving when you told me you hadn't done part of your homework?

P: (*Nods.*)

T: What's the evidence that I would frown and be disapproving? . . . Do you have any evidence on the other side? [The therapist shows the patient how to use the questions at the bottom of the Dysfunctional Thought Record to evaluate her spontaneous image.]

In another situation, the therapist teaches the patient to compare a spontaneous image with what is really happening.

P: I was in the library late last night, and I had an image of the building being real deserted, and then I saw myself suddenly feeling really sick and passing out and having no one there to help me.

T: Was it true that the library was completely deserted?

P: No. It was getting late, near closing time, but there were still a few people around.

T: Okay. With this kind of image, when you're spontaneously imagining something happening right at the moment, you can do a reality check. You can ask yourself, "Is the library deserted? Am I actually feeling sick now?" If you had known to do that last night, what do you think would have happened to your mood?

P: I'd have felt less nervous.

In general, it is preferable to use techniques in imagery form when dealing with images rather than the verbal techniques suggested in this section because images tend to respond better to imagery-based interventions. However, a patient who has many vivid, distressing images will benefit from a variety of techniques and sometimes the verbal technique of doing a reality check is helpful.

Repeating the Image

The repetition technique is often useful when the patient clearly is imagining an exaggerated, though noncatastrophic, outcome. The therapist suggests that the patient keep imagining the original image over and over again and pay attention to whether the image and her level of distress change. Some patients seem to do an automatic reality check and envision each succeeding image more realistically and with less dysphoria.

T: Okay, Sally, so you had the image of asking your professor for an extension, and he clearly got quite upset, yelling at you, bending over close to you, waving his hands wildly saying, "How dare you! You knew when it was due. I can't believe you're asking for this! Get out! Get out!"

P: Yes.

T: I wonder, could you imagine this again? Start out the same way. See what happens.

P: (*Closes eyes.*)

T: Finished? What happened?

P: He was pretty upset. He still yelled at me, told me to get out.

T: This time did he wave his hands, bend over too close to you?

P: No. He just stood up and stiffened his arms on his desk.

T: Okay. Do the same thing again.

The therapist has Sally repeat the scene three or four times. By the last repetition, her image has changed quite a bit: The professor is leaning back in his chair, gives Sally an annoyed look and says no in an unkindly but nonthreatening way. Sally's anxiety diminishes significantly.

Substituting, Stopping, and Distracting Oneself from Images

These three techniques have been extensively described elsewhere. They are designed to bring quick relief from images but generally result in little or no cognitive restructuring.

Image stopping is analogous to thought stopping (Davis, Eshelman, & McKay, 1988) and may be used alone or followed by image substitution or distraction. Here the patient recognizes a distressing image and then tries to cut it off. She may, for example, imagine a stop sign and perhaps yell, "Stop!" inside her head whenever the image appears. She may also try snapping a rubberband around her wrist, clapping her hands loudly, or engaging in some other behavior incompatible with continuing to hold the distressing image in mind. Distraction and refocusing techniques (described in Chapter 12 in relation to automatic thoughts) may be used as well.

T: To summarize, Sally, sometimes when you notice a distressing image, it's too inconvenient or too difficult to work on it at the time. That's when you might try image stopping or distraction. Can we practice it now? Can you get that distressing image you told me about before in your mind again? Which technique do you want to try?

Substituting a more pleasant image has also been extensively described elsewhere (Beck & Emery, 1985). It, too, must be regularly practiced in order for the patient to experience relief from distressing spontaneous images.

T: Sally, another way of dealing with this kind of distressing image is to substitute a different image. Some people like to imagine that the distressing image is a picture on a television set. Then they imagine changing the channel to a different scene, like lying on a beach, or walking through the woods, or remembering a pleasant memory from the past. Would you like to try this technique? We'll first have you picture the pleasant scene in as much detail as possible, using as many senses as possible, then I'll have you practice switching from a distressing image to the pleasant one. . . . Now what pleasant scene would you like to imagine?

Pairing pleasant imagery with relaxation exercises is another option. Patients often experience relief by inducing a pleasant image when their initial distress is low to moderate but not high.

REVIEWING TECHNIQUES FOR RESPONDING TO SPONTANEOUS IMAGERY

Having taught the patient one or two strategies to deal with spontaneous images, the therapist maximizes the probability that she will practice them.

T: Sally, let's quickly review what you've learned so far about responding to your images, and maybe you could write a few things down?

P: Yeah.

T: You won't really know in advance which technique is going to help. But if you have a written list, you're more likely to keep trying until you find what *does* help. In the next couple of sessions I can teach you some more techniques if it looks like it'd be helpful. We'll keep practicing together here and you can practice at home until you get really good at the techniques. Then I think you'll find that you feel more in control of the images and of how they affect you emotionally.

INDUCING IMAGERY AS A THERAPEUTIC TOOL

At times, the therapist seeks to *induce* an image as opposed to helping the patient respond to a spontaneous image. Covert rehearsal to uncover obstacles related to homework (see Chapter 14) is an example. Three other induced imaginal techniques are described next.

Rehearsal of Coping Techniques

The therapist uses this technique in session to help the patient mentally practice coping strategies in her imagination. This technique differs from "coping in the image" because here the therapist *induces* an image to practice cognitive therapy techniques rather than having the patient imagine how she will cope more broadly in a spontaneous image.

T: Okay, you're predicting that you're going to have a rough time giving the oral report in class.

P: Yeah.

T: How about if we have you imagine yourself coping with it? When will you first notice your anxiety going up?

P: When I wake up.

T: And what will be going through your mind?

P: I'm going to mess up. And I'll picture myself stammering and stuttering and being unable to talk.

T: You mean in class?

P: Yeah.

T: Okay, what could you do?

P: Tell myself to relax. Remind myself I've practiced this report a lot.

T: Okay, what then?

P: I could do some controlled breathing. That relaxes me some.

T: Okay, can you see yourself doing that?

P: Yeah.

T: Then what?

P: I feel a little better but I'm still too nervous for breakfast. I just shower, get dressed, get ready to go.

T: What's going through your mind?

P: What if I keep getting more and more nervous?

T: How about imagining yourself reading the coping card we made before on the way to class? Can you imagine pulling it out and reading it?

P: Yeah . . . I guess it helps some.

T: As you get near class, how about if you imagine jumping ahead in time. You've finished the talk, and now you're sitting there listening to someone else. . . . How do you feel now?

P: Some relief. Still worried, but not as bad.

T: Okay, now you're walking into class. What happens next and what do you do?

The patient continues imagining herself realistically coping with the situation in detail. Then she writes down the specific techniques she predicts will help.

Distancing

Distancing is another induced imagery technique to reduce distress and help patients see a problem in greater perspective. In the following example, the therapist helps the patient see that her difficulties are likely to be time-limited and thereby gives her hope.

T: Sally, I know you're feeling kind of hopeless now and you're predicting that these problems will go on and on. Do you think it would help if you could envision getting through this rough period?

P: I guess. It's hard to imagine.

T: Well, let's see. How about if you try to picture yourself next semester. It's your sophomore year, let's say, midway through the fall; you'll still be in college?

P: Probably.

T: Any idea what life is like?

P: I don't know. It's hard for me to think that far ahead.

T: Well, let's be concrete. When do you wake up? Where are you?

P: Probably I wake up around 8:00 or 8:30. I guess I'm in an off-campus apartment.

T: Living alone?

P: Maybe in a house with other students, some people from my floor this year. We've been talking about it.

T: Okay, you wake up. What happens next?

P: I probably rush off to class. It'll take longer to get there if I'm not in a dorm.

T: Do you see any of your housemates before you go? Do you go to class alone or with one of them?

P: I don't know.

T: Well, it's your image. You decide.

P: Okay, I guess I'd walk over with one of them.

T: What do you talk about on the way—or are you silent?

P: Oh no, we'd be talking about school or people we know. Something like that.

T: Then what?

P: Go to class.

T: A big lecture hall like most of your classes this year?

P: No, probably not, classes should be smaller next year.

T: And what do you want to imagine happens in class? Do you interact or are you quiet?

P: Well, hopefully by then I'd know more people. I'd feel more comfortable. I'd probably still be quiet, but I might be participating more.

T: How do you feel when you imagine this scene?

P: Good.

T: How would you feel about finishing out this scene for homework? Then every time you have the thought, "I'll never get out of this," you could try switching to this scene to see if it has any effect on your mood.

P: I'll try.

T: Now is this just the power of positive thinking, imagining this scene? Or could you really do some things to make it happen? In fact, aren't you already doing things to make it happen?

P: That's true.

Another distancing technique helps a patient deal with the imagined aftermath of a catastrophe. Marie, described previously, fears that her children would be devastated forever if she died. Her therapist has her imagine their realistic level of distress at different points in time, instead of just immediately after the accident. (This technique is similar to jumping ahead in time; it involves the passage of *years*, though, instead of minutes, hours, or days.)

T: Marie, who do you imagine breaks the news of your death to the kids?

P: My husband.

T: How does he do it?

P: (*Sobbing.*) He puts his arms around them. He says, "There's been an accident. Mommy's gone."

T: And then?

P: They don't believe it, not really, at first. They start crying and saying, "No, it's not true. I want Mommy."

T: They're feeling pretty bad?

P: Yeah. Real bad.

T: . . . (*Waits a moment.*) Can you jump ahead some? It's now 6 months later. What's going on now? Can you see them?

P: They're in school. Looking real sad. Bewildered. Kind of empty.

T: How bad are they feeling?

P: Still pretty bad.

T: Can we jump ahead 2 years? How old are they now?

P: Melissa, she's 8. Linda, she's 6.

T: What are they doing?

P: Playing outside. It's our house. I don't think my husband would move.

T: What are they doing?

P: Playing with the next door neighbors. Jump rope or throwing a ball or something.

T: How are they feeling now?

P: Okay, when they don't think about me.

T: And when they do?

P: (*Tears up.*) They still cry sometimes. It's confusing.

T: As bad as when they first found out?

P: No, not that bad.

The therapist gently leads Marie through a succession of images, 5, 10, and 20 years after her imagined death. Through this exercise, Marie is able to see that the initial devastation her daughters feel eventually subsides to briefer periods of sadness and grief with which they are able to cope. Imagining in detail that her daughters grow up and create new families of their own significantly reduces Marie's fear of her own death in an automobile accident.

Reduction of Perceived Threat

A third type of induced image is designed to allow the patient to view a situation with a more realistic assessment of actual threat. For example, the therapist encourages Sally to modify her image of her class presentation by imagining the encouraging faces of her friends in the room. Pam, a patient who feared undergoing a Caesarean section, envisioned all the life-saving equipment in the delivery room and the caring faces of the nurse and doctor behind their masks.

In summary many, if not most, patients experience automatic thoughts in the form of spontaneous images. Persistent (though nonintrusive) questioning is often required to help patients recognize their images. Patients who do have frequent, distressing images benefit from regular practice of several imagery techniques. In addition, images may be induced for various therapeutic purposes.

Chapter 14

HOMEWORK

Homework is an integral, not optional, part of cognitive therapy (Beck et al., 1979). In essence, the therapist seeks to extend the opportunities for cognitive and behavioral change *throughout the patient's week*. Good homework assignments provide opportunities for the patient to educate herself further (e.g., through bibliotherapy), to collect data (e.g., through monitoring her thoughts, feelings, and behavior), to test her thoughts and beliefs, to modify her thinking, to practice cognitive and behavioral tools, and to experiment with new behaviors. Homework can maximize what was learned in a therapy session and lead to an increase in the patient's sense of self-efficacy.

A number of researchers have found that cognitive therapy patients who carry out homework assignments progress better in therapy than those who do not (e.g., Neimeyer & Feixas, 1990; Persons et al., 1988). Many patients do homework quite willingly and easily; a few do not. It is important to note that even the most experienced therapists encounter difficulty with an occasional patient who, despite careful preparation, rarely does any *written* assignments. Nevertheless, the therapist should initially assume that any given patient *will* do homework if it has been set up properly. The therapist takes care, for example, to tailor assignments to the individual, provide a sound rationale, uncover potential obstacles, and modify relevant beliefs to enhance the probability that patients will comply. This chapter is divided into four parts: setting homework assignments, increasing the likelihood of successful completion of homework, conceptualizing problems, and reviewing completed homework.

SETTING HOMEWORK ASSIGNMENTS

There is no set formula for assigning homework. Rather, homework is tailored to the individual patient, set collaboratively, and devised according to the content and goals of the session, the patient's and therapist's overall goals of therapy, and the therapist's conceptualization of the patient and the patient's stage of therapy. When suggesting homework assignments, the therapist should, of course, take into consideration individual characteristics of the patient: her reading and writing abilities, her motivation and willingness to comply with homework, her level of distress and cognitive functioning, and practical constraints (e.g., of time), to name a few.

Generally the therapist takes the lead in suggesting homework assignments in the first stage of therapy. Gradually, as with agenda setting, however, the therapist begins to ask the patient to devise her own assignments (e.g., "Now that we've finished talking about this problem with your roommate, what do you think would be helpful for you to do this week?"). Patients who routinely set their own homework by the end of therapy are more likely to continue doing so when therapy is over.

In this first section, typical assignments are presented. Ongoing homework assignments are described; other tasks appropriate for initial, middle, and final phases of therapy are delineated. Then a sample of Sally's homework assignments is provided. The final portion of this section offers guidelines for selection of assignments.

Ongoing Homework Assignments

Typical ongoing homework assignments are discussed below.

1. *Behavioral activation* is especially important for inactive patients but may also be quite helpful to many patients whose goal is either to resume previous activities or to enrich their lives through experimenting with new activities. Activity scheduling can be accomplished in the more formal manner presented in Chapter 12 or in a casual way (e.g., "Any activities from your goal list you'd either like to try or to find out more information about this week?").

A second type of behavioral activity follows logically from the session content, consisting of practicing new skills and/or implementing solutions emanating from practical problem-solving. Sally, for example, had some problems with her roommate. Following discussion and role-play in the session, Sally agreed to try to negotiate issues such as noise and clutter with her roommate. Direct problem-solving with successful behavioral follow-through often provides an important boost in mood.

2. *Monitoring automatic thoughts* is an important assignment from the first session forward. As described in Chapter 3, the patient asks herself, "What's going through my mind right now?" whenever she notices her mood changing. Initially she may jot down these thoughts on paper, in a notebook, or on an index card. As soon as it is appropriate, the therapist

teaches her to write automatic thoughts on a Dysfunctional Thought Record.

The therapist advises the patient that monitoring automatic thoughts can actually lead to an *increase* in distress unless the patient also tries to respond adaptively to her cognitions. For this reason, therapist and patient might compose coping cards (see Chapter 12) to be read at home which address predicted distressing thoughts.

3. *Bibliotherapy* is another useful ongoing assignment. It is usually valuable to have the patient both read and note her reactions: what she agreed with, disagreed with, and had questions about. (See Appendix C for a suggested patient reading list.)

4. *Reviewing the past therapy session* helps consolidate learning. Such a review might consist of reading notes written during the session itself (or immediately afterward) and/or listening to an audiotape of the therapy session. While listening to the tape, the patient might write down the main points of or conclusions drawn in the session, or she might record the automatic thoughts and dysfunctional beliefs and adaptive responses identified in the session. An alternative to taping and listening to the entire session is to record only a summary of the session made during the last few minutes of the session. As the therapist may wish to have his own audiotape to review between sessions (see Chapter 18), he may ask the patient to supply her own tapes and recording equipment.

5. *Preparing for the next therapy session* is natural for many patients and does not require a specific ongoing assignment. These patients automatically collect their thoughts in anticipation of the therapist's standard format of questioning at the beginning of each session. Some patients, however, avoid thinking about therapy between sessions or have difficulty condensing the important items they want to talk about into a few sentences. It is useful to have these patients make mental or written notes prior to each session. The Session Bridging Worksheet (Chapter 4, Figure 4.1) can be a useful guide.

Additional Assignments

The assignments just described may be useful for each session. In addition, the therapist should evaluate the utility of other assignments that may be appropriate for a limited number of sessions. During the initial session, for example, it is often helpful to have the patient refine her goal list (see Chapter 3) and start a positive self-statement log (see Chapter 12). During the next few sessions, homework may emphasize evaluating and responding to automatic thoughts.

When underlying assumptions and beliefs are identified, the patient may find it useful to review a completed Cognitive Conceptualization

Diagram (Chapter 10). Having begun to restructure dysfunctional beliefs in session, the patient may continue working on Core Belief Worksheets (Chapter 11) at home. Either prior to or following belief modification, the patient may experiment with continuing behavioral change: practicing newly acquired skills (such as assertiveness), acting "as if" (see Chapter 10), and testing thoughts and beliefs through behavioral experiments (see Chapters 10 and 12).

Finally, homework in the final phase of therapy may be oriented toward termination and relapse prevention (see Chapter 15): organizing therapy notes, responding to automatic thoughts about termination, and developing plans for predicted future difficulties.

Although the assignments listed next are appropriate for many patients, it is important to realize that a great number of homework tasks are individualized, designed especially for a particular patient.

A Sampling of Homework Assignments for Sally

Session 1
1. Refine goal list.
2. When my mood changes, ask myself, "What's going through my mind right now?" and jot down thoughts (and images). Remind myself that these thoughts may or may not be true.
3. Remind myself that I'm *depressed* right now, not lazy, and that's why things are hard.
4. Think about what I want to put on the agenda next week (what problem or situation) and how to name it.
5. Read booklet (*Coping with Depression*; see Appendix D) and therapy notes.
6. Go swimming or running three times this week.

Session 2
1. When I notice my mood changing, ask myself, "What's going through my mind right now?" and jot down automatic thoughts (which may or may not be completely true). Try to do this at least once a day.
2. If I cannot figure out my automatic thoughts, jot down just the situation. Remember, learning to identify my thinking is a skill I will get better at, like typing.
3. Ask Ron for help with Chapter 5 of econ book.
4. Read over therapy notes once a day.
5. Continue swimming/running. Plan three activities with roommate.

Session 3
1. Read therapy notes once a day.
2. Continue running/swimming/activities with Jane.
3. Ask Lisa to study for chem exam with me.
4. Add to credit list (positive self-statement log).
5. Fill out first four columns of Dysfunctional Thought Record (DTR) once a day when my mood gets worse and use questions at bottom to think of response.

Session 4
1. Write down automatic thoughts on the DTR.
2. Review therapy notes.
3. Fill in activity monitor as much as possible.
4. Discuss/negotiate with roommate about noise in late evening.
5. Keep a credit list (positive self-statement log).

Session 5
1. Fill out first four columns of the DTR when mood changes and mentally use questions at bottom to develop an alternative response.
2. Read therapy notes.
3. Follow through on activities scheduled in session.
4. Credit list.
5. Approach teaching assistant for extra help.

Session 6
1. Complete DTRs when distressed.
2. Read therapy notes (once a day).
3. Credit list.
4. Read coping card when anxious about lit paper.
5. Continue scheduling of activities.

Session 7
1. DTR.
2. Read therapy notes.
3. Credit list.
4. Ask one or two questions after class.
5. Read coping cards three times a day and as needed.

Session 8
1. DTR.
2. Read therapy notes and coping cards as needed.
3. Credit list.
4. Ask one or two questions in class.
5. Read over Case Conceptualization Diagram.

Session 9
1. DTR.
2. Read therapy notes and coping cards, one to three times a day.
3. Answer one or two questions or make a comment in class (economics and chemistry).
4. Do bottom of Core Belief Worksheet.
5. Bring up noise problems with roommate.
6. Go to Dr. Smith during office hours.
7. Advantages–disadvantages of Philadelphia versus home for summer.

Session 12 (Penultimate Session)
1. DTR about termination.
2. Organize therapy notes from beginning.
3. Review notes on doing a self-therapy session.

INCREASING THE LIKELIHOOD
OF SUCCESSFUL HOMEWORK

Although some patients easily do the suggested assignments, homework is more problematic for others. Implementation of the following guidelines increases the likelihood that the patient will be successful with homework and experience an elevation in mood:

1. Tailor the assignment to the individual. (Be 90–100% sure the patient can and will do the assignment.) Err on the side of devising assignments that are too easy rather than too hard.
2. Provide a rationale as to how and why the assignment might help.
3. Set homework collaboratively; seek the patient's input and agreement.
4. Make homework a no-lose proposition.
5. Begin the assignment (when possible) in session.
6. Help set up systems for remembering to do the assignment.
7. Anticipate possible problems; do covert rehearsal when indicated.
8. Prepare for a possible negative outcome (when applicable).

Tailoring Homework to the Individual

Successful completion of homework can speed up therapy and lead to an increased sense of mastery and improved mood. Homework should, therefore, be carefully considered to maximize the probability of success. Rather than suggesting assignments according to a prescribed formula, the therapist should take into consideration the patient's characteristics (mentioned in the introduction to this chapter) and desires.

Joan, for example, was a patient who did not grasp the cognitive model in the first session and, indeed, became slightly irritated when her (novice) therapist kept pushing her to identify her automatic thoughts. She told her therapist, "You don't understand; I don't *know* what is going through my mind at the time; all I know is that I'm very upset." A homework assignment to jot down her automatic thoughts would have been inappropriate for this session. A second patient, Barbara, on the other hand, had already read a popular book on cognitive therapy and had an unusually good grasp of her automatic thoughts. Her initial homework assignment was to complete the first four columns of the Dysfunctional Thought Record whenever she became upset.

While the type of assignment is important, so is the *amount* of homework. Sally was a motivated patient who was "in sync" with homework as she was still a student. She was easily able to accomplish more at home than Joan who was more severely depressed and had been out of school for many years.

A third step in tailoring homework to the individual patient involves breaking down assignments into manageable steps. Examples include reading one chapter of a layman's cognitive therapy book or school textbook, doing the first four columns of a Dysfunctional Thought Record, spending 10 to 15 minutes paying bills, doing just two loads of laundry, and driving to the nearby supermarket but not going in initially.

It is important to predict potential difficulties before assigning homework. This can be done by considering the patient's diagnosis and presenting problems. The severely depressed patient, for example, will probably benefit more from behavioral (as opposed to cognitive) tasks initially. The avoidant patient, on the other hand, will probably shy away from behavioral assignments which she perceives as challenging and capable of evoking dysphoria. A patient who is feeling anxious and overwhelmed might feel incapable of doing *any* assignment if the therapist suggests too many tasks for her to do. It is thus far better to err on the side of providing homework assignments that are a little too easy. Failure to carry out an assignment, or to do it properly, often leads a patient to feel self-critical or hopeless.

Providing a Rationale

Patients are more likely to comply with homework assignments if they understand the reason for doing them. Sally's therapist, for example, introduced a homework suggestion in the following way: "Sally, do you think it would be helpful for both of us if we knew a little better how you're spending your time? Then, we can see if you're overloaded with one type of activity and perhaps not spending enough time on other things."

The therapist usually provides a brief rationale initially; later in therapy, he encourages the patient to think about the purpose of an assignment, for example, "Sally, what would be the point of checking with your roommate about her plans for this weekend?" "Why might it be a good idea to continue keeping the credit list?" It is also useful to point out to patients that they may feel better *faster* if they make the effort to do homework: "The research shows that people who do therapy homework generally seem to make better progress than people who don't." It is also important to stress the rationale for doing homework *daily*. Changing one's thinking and behavior requires ongoing attention and effort.

Setting Homework Collaboratively

The therapist ensures that the patient not only understands the rationale for an assignment but also *agrees* to do it: "Sally, what do you think about asking your professor a question after class?" Overly compliant patients may readily agree to homework in session but fail to complete it. When the therapist sees such a pattern developing, he takes a few extra steps, such as asking the following sorts of questions: "How likely is it, do you think, that you'll be able to fill out the Dysfunctional Thought Record a couple of times this week?" "Is this something you really think will help?" "Would you prefer to do it mentally this week, and we can fill it out together at our next session?" "How could we set it up so you'd be more likely to do it?"

As therapy progresses, the therapist encourages the patient to set her own assignments. "What would you like to do this week, vis-à-vis [this problem]?" "What could you do this week if you start getting uncomfortably anxious?" "How will you handle [this problem] if it does arise?"

Making Homework a No-Lose Proposition

As mentioned in Chapter 3, it is helpful when setting up assignments initially to stress that useful data can be obtained even if the patient does fail to complete her homework. In this way, the patient who does not do the homework is less likely to brand herself a failure and thus feel more dysphoric.

THERAPIST: Sally, if you get all this homework done, that's good. But, if you have trouble doing it, that's okay, especially if you can figure out what thoughts are getting in your way. So, either you'll do the assignments, or see if you can mentally keep track of what's going through your mind that keeps you from doing them. Then, we can talk about those thoughts next week; they'll be important information for us. Okay?

Sometimes patients fail to do a significant portion of their homework for 2 weeks in a row, or they do it immediately before the therapy session instead of daily. In these cases, the therapist should uncover the psychological and/or practical obstacles that got in the way and stress how essential homework is, instead of continuing to make it a no-lose proposition.

Starting Homework in the Session

Especially in the first stage of therapy, it is advisable to allow time in the therapy session for the patient to begin an assignment. Doing so is useful to the therapist so he can gauge whether the assignment is at an appropriate level of difficulty. It is also useful to the patient, who is more likely to continue an assignment than to initiate one. This is especially critical because patients often describe the hardest part of doing homework as the period *just before* they start it—that is, motivating themselves to get started.

Remembering to Do Homework

It is critically important to socialize patients from the very beginning to write down what their assignments are in session. Several other strategies are useful for patients who nevertheless forget to carry them out. They can be instructed to pair an assignment with another daily activity (e.g., "How about pulling out the activity schedule at meal times and right before bed?"). They can post notes on their refrigerator, their bathroom mirror, or the dashboard of their car. A discussion of how they remember to take medication or give it to others can prompt them to recall previously used techniques. Straightforward problem-solving is often indicated; for example, figuring out together that the patient could listen to therapy tapes in the car on the way to and from work.

Anticipating Problems

It is important for the therapist to put himself in the patient's shoes, considering the following:

> Is the amount of homework reasonable for this patient?
> Is the degree of difficulty appropriate?
> Does it seem overwhelming?
> Does it seem logically related to her goals?
> How likely is she to do it?
> What practical problems may get in the way (time, energy, opportunity)?
> What thoughts may get in the way?

The therapist asks the patient how likely (0–100%) she is to do an assignment. If the therapist is not 90–100% confident that the patient can and will do an assignment, he should consider one or more of the following strategies:

1. *Covert rehearsal*, illustrated below, uses induced imagery to uncover and solve potential homework-related problems.

T: Sally, do you think anything will get in the way of your going to the teaching assistant for help?

PATIENT: I'm not sure.

T: When would be a good time to go? (*getting her to specify and commit to a time.*)

P: Friday morning, I guess. That's when his office hours are.

T: Can you imagine it's Friday morning right now? Can you picture it? Can you imagine saying to yourself, "I really should go to the TA's office"?

P: Yeah.

T: Where are you? (*Asking for details so patient will more easily be able to visualize the scene and accurately identify her thoughts and emotions.*)

P: In my room.

T: Doing what?

P: Well, I just finished getting dressed.

T: And how are you feeling?

P: A little nervous, I guess.

T: And what's going through your mind?

P: I don't want to go. Maybe I'll just read the chapter again myself.

T: And how are you going to answer that thought?

P: I don't know. It sounds good to me. (*Laughs.*)

T: Do you want to remind yourself that this would be a good experiment to test your prediction that you won't be able to understand the material even if you get help?

P: I suppose so.

T: Would it help to read a coping card?

P: Probably. [The therapist and patient jointly compose a coping card as described in Chapter 12.]

T: Okay. Now can you imagine you're dressed and you're thinking, "I'll just read the chapter myself instead of going." Now what happens?

P: I think, "Wait a minute. This is supposed to be an experiment. Now where's that coping card?"

T: Oh, where is it?

P: Knowing me, I'd have to look for it.

T: Is there someplace you could put it as soon as you get back today?

P: I don't exactly want my roommate to see it. . . . Maybe in the bottom drawer of my desk.

T: Okay. Can you imagine pulling out the card and reading it?

P: Yeah.

T: Now, what happens?

P: Probably I remember why I *should* go, but I still don't want to. So, I decide to clean my room first.

T: What could you remind yourself at this point?

P: That I may as well go and get it over with. That maybe it really will help. That if I stop and clean I may end up not going at all.

T: Good. Then what happens?

P: I go.

T: And then?

P: I get there. I ask him the question. I don't understand it all. I tell him what I'm confused about. He probably helps.

T: And how do you feel at this point?

P: Pretty good. I'm glad I went.

This covert rehearsal of homework helps patient and therapist discover which practical obstacles and dysfunctional thoughts may hinder the completion of homework.

2. *Suggesting a different assignment* may be indicated if the therapist judges that an assignment *is* inappropriate or if covert rehearsal has not been sufficiently effective. It is far better to substitute an easier homework assignment which the patient is more likely to do than to have her establish the habit of not doing what she had agreed to in session.

T: Sally, I'm not sure you're ready to do this. [Or, "I'm not sure this assignment is appropriate."] What do you think? Do you want to go ahead and try or wait until another time?"

3. *A rational–emotional role-play* may help motivate a reluctant patient when the therapist judges it is quite important for a patient to do a given assignment. (As described in Chapter 10, this technique is not used early in therapy as it can be perceived as somewhat challenging.)

T: I'm still not sure you'll actually pull out the coping card to get you going.

P: Probably not.

T: Okay, how about if we do a rational–emotional role-play about this? We've done this before. I'll be the intellectual part of you; you be the emotional part. You argue as hard as you can against me so I can see all the arguments you're using not to read your coping cards and start studying. You start.

P: Okay. I don't feel like doing this.

T: It's true that I don't feel like doing it, but that's irrelevant. It doesn't matter if I feel like it or not. It's what I *need* to do.

P: But, I can do it later.

T: True, but my usual pattern is *not* to do it later. I don't want to reinforce a bad habit by putting it off. Here I have the opportunity to strengthen a new, better habit.

P: But it won't matter this one time.

T: True. Any one individual time isn't all that crucial. On the other hand, I'll be better off in the long run if I strengthen this good habit as much as I can.

P: I don't know, I just don't want to.

T: I don't have to pay attention to what I *want* to do now or *don't* want to do now. In the long run, I *want* to do things that I need to do to reach my goals and feel good about myself, and I *don't* want to constantly avoid things I don't feel like doing.

P: . . . I've run out of arguments.

T: Okay. Let's switch parts, then we'll get some of it down in writing [or talk about listening to this part of the tape].

Following role reversal, the therapist has another choice point. He may collaboratively reassign the original homework task (e.g., "How do you feel *now* about trying [this assignment]?"). If they do decide to keep the assignment, they may jointly write a coping card with some points mentioned in the role-play above. If the therapist believes it is unlikely that the patient will fulfill the assignment, however, he suggests a change in homework rather than risk the patient's feeling like a failure if she does not do it.

Preparing for a Possible Negative Outcome

When devising a behavioral experiment or testing an assumption, it is important to set up a scenario that is likely to be successful. For example, Sally and her therapist discussed which professor was more likely to be receptive to questions after class, what words she might use when negotiating late-night noise with her roommate, and how much help was reasonable to ask from her neighbor. If the therapist believes that a behavioral experiment might not turn out as well as expected, he might help the patient do some advance responding to predicted automatic thoughts (see Chapter 12).

T: Now I suppose it *could* happen that your neighbor says he can't help you. If that happens, what will go through your mind?

P: That I shouldn't have asked. That he probably thinks I'm stupid for asking.

T: What other reasons might he have for saying no? (*Seeking an alternative explanation.*)

P: That he was too busy.

T: Uh huh.

P: (*Thinks.*)

T: Might it be that he doesn't understand the material well enough to explain it to you? Or, that he simply doesn't like tutoring? Or, that he's preoccupied with something else?

P: I guess so.

T: Do you have any evidence so far that he thinks you're stupid?

P: No, but we did disagree about politics.

T: And did you get the idea that he thought your ideas were definitely stupid or that you simply had another point of view?

P: That we just felt differently about it.

T: So, as far as you know, he doesn't view you as stupid?

P: No, I don't think so.

T: So even if he turns you down, it won't *necessarily* be that he's changed his view of you, based on your request for help?

P: No, I guess not.

T: Okay, we've agreed that you'll approach him later today and ask for help. Either he'll help you, and that's good, or he'll say no, and then what will you remind yourself?

P: That it doesn't mean he thinks I'm stupid. He may just be busy or unsure of the stuff himself or not like to tutor people.

Advance discussion of a potential problem guards against possible demoralization when the patient criticizes herself.

CONCEPTUALIZING DIFFICULTIES

If the patient has difficulty doing her homework, the therapist uses this problem as an opportunity to understand the patient better. The therapist considers whether the failure to do homework was related to a practical problem, a psychological problem, a psychological problem masked as a practical problem, and/or a problem related to the *therapist's* cognitions.

Practical Problems

Most practical problems can be avoided if the therapist carefully sets the assignment and prepares the patient to do it. Covert rehearsal (as described above) can also ferret out potential difficulties. Four common practical problems and their remedies are described next.

Doing Therapy Homework at the Last Minute

Ideally, patients carry on the work of the therapy session *throughout the week*. For example, it is most useful for patients to catch and record their automatic thoughts at the moment they notice their mood changing and to respond to these thoughts either mentally or in writing. Some patients avoid thinking about therapy between sessions. Often, this avoidance is part of a larger problem, and therapist and patient may first have to identify and modify certain beliefs (e.g., "If I focus on a problem instead of distracting myself, I'll only feel worse"; or "I can't change, so why even try?"). Other patients, however, need only a gentle reminder not to do homework only at the last minute: "Some patients do their homework the night before the session. How useful do you think it would be for *you* to do it the night before the session as opposed to all through the week?"

Forgetting the Rationale for an Assignment

Occasionally, a patient neglects an assignment because she does not remember *why* she was asked to do it. This problem can be avoided by having a patient (who has demonstrated this difficulty) record the rationale next to an assignment.

P: I didn't do the relaxation exercises [or read the coping cards or practice controlled breathing or record my activities] because I was feeling fine this week.

T: Do you remember what we said a few weeks ago—why it's helpful to practice this every week, regardless of how you're feeling?

P: I'm not sure.

T: Well, let's say you don't practice your relaxation exercises for 3 weeks. Then you have a very stressful week. How sharp will your skills be then?

P: Not as sharp as if I had practiced every week, I guess.

T: Could we have you write down relaxation exercises for homework again this week? Any other problems with practicing them? And maybe you'll want to add why it is you've decided to practice them, even if you're feeling well.

Disorganization

For patients who continue to have difficulty organizing themselves or remembering to do homework, it is advisable to set up a special structure or regimen for doing so. One technique is the use of a homework monitor, a simple diagram the therapist can draw in session. The patient is simply instructed to check off each assignment as she completes it.

Another technique is to ask the patient to get a calendar or appoint-

	W	Th	F	Sat	Sun	M	T
1. Read therapy notes							
2. Credit list							
3. Do a DTR							
4. Ask a question in class							

ment book. The therapist can ask her to write down what her assignments are in each day's space. (They might do the first day together in the office and the patient might be asked to write down the rest in the reception room after the session.) Later, after completing an assignment, the patient can cross it off.

A third technique is to ask the patient to call the therapist's office and leave a message when she has completed an assignment. Knowing that her therapist is expecting a message may motivate her to do the homework.

These techniques, as with any intervention, should be suggested with a rationale and collaboratively agreed upon.

Difficulty with an Assignment

If the therapist realizes at a subsequent session that a homework assignment has been too difficult or ill-defined (common problems with novice therapists), he should take care to offer this explanation to the patient (who may have unfairly criticized *herself* for not having successfully completed an assignment).

T: Sally, now that we've talked about the problem you had with the homework, I can see that I didn't explain it well enough to you [or, I can see that it wasn't really appropriate]. What went through your mind when you couldn't [or didn't] do it?

Here the therapist has an opportunity to (1) model that he can make and admit to a mistake, (2) build rapport, (3) demonstrate to the patient that he *is* concerned with tailoring therapy—and homework assignments—to her, and (4) help the patient see an alternative explanation for her lack of success.

Psychological Problems

Given that an assignment was properly set up and the patient had the opportunity to do it, difficulty in completing it may have stemmed from one of the psychological factors described next.

Negative Predictions

When patients are in psychological distress and particularly when they are depressed, they tend to assume negative outcomes. To identify dysfunctional cognitions that interfered with doing a homework assignment, the therapist has the patient recall a *specific* time she thought about doing the assignment and then explores related cognitions and feelings:

T: Was there a time this week when you *did* think about reading the pamphlet on depression?

P: Yes. I thought about it on and off.

T: Tell me about one of these times. Did you think about it last night, for example?

P: Yeah. I was going to do it after dinner.

T: What happened?

P: I don't know. I just couldn't make myself do it.

T: How were you feeling?

P: Down, sad, tired.

T: What was going through your mind as you thought about reading the pamphlet?

P: This is hard. I probably won't be able to concentrate. I won't understand it.

T: Sounds like you were feeling pretty low. No wonder you were having trouble getting started. I wonder, though, how we could test this idea that you won't be able to concentrate and understand it.

P: I guess I could try it.

The patient might then conduct an experiment right in session. Following a successful outcome, she might write down her conclusions; for example, "Sometimes my thoughts are inaccurate and I can do more than I think. Next time I feel hopeless, I can do an experiment to test my ideas." (Note: If the experiment were unsuccessful, the therapist would change the assignment to a more basic task.)

Other negative predictions, such as "My roommate won't want to go to that meeting with me," or "I won't understand the material even if I ask for help," or "Doing homework will make me feel worse," can be behaviorally tested in a straightforward manner (though the therapist might again consider preparing the patient in advance for her reaction to a possible negative outcome). Other thoughts, such as "I can't do anything right," or "I might fail this course," might be evaluated with standard questions (see Chapter 8) and alternative responses developed.

If the patient reveals ambivalence about doing an assignment, it is important for the therapist to acknowledge that he does not know what the outcome will be: "I don't know for sure that doing this assignment *will* help. What will you lose if it doesn't work? What's the potential gain in the long run if it does work?" Alternatively, patient and therapist could list advantages and disadvantages of doing the homework. If the patient has difficulty identifying her thoughts about homework or has difficulty honestly expressing them to the therapist, she might be asked to fill out a form designed to specify homework problems (see Appendix D).

Finally, a patient may benefit from work at the belief level. Homework may activate beliefs such as these:

> "I'm inadequate/helpless/incompetent."
> "Doing therapy homework means I'm defective."
> "I shouldn't have to put forth so much effort to feel better."
> "My therapist is trying to control me."
> "If I think about my problems, I'll feel worse and worse."

Beliefs such as these can be identified and modified through techniques described in Chapters 10 and 11.

Overestimating the Demands of an Assignment

Some patients overestimate how inconvenient or difficult it will be to do homework or do not realize that doing a therapy assignment will be time-limited.

T: What could get in the way of your doing a Dysfunctional Thought Record a few times this week?

P: I'm not sure I'll find the time.

T: How long do you think it will take each time?

P: Not that long. Maybe 10 minutes. But, I'm pretty rushed these days, you know. I do have a million things to do.

Patient and therapist then do straightforward problem-solving to find possible time slots. Alternatively, the therapist can propose an analogy, stressing that the inconvenience of doing assignments is time-limited:

T: It certainly is true; you *are* very busy these days. I wonder, what would you do if you had to take time every day to do something that would save your life [or your child's/significant other's/family member's life]? What would happen, for example, if you needed a blood transfusion every day?

P: Well, of course I'd find the time.

T: Now, it's obviously not life-threatening if you don't do this assignment, but the principle is the same. In a minute, we can talk specifically about how you could cut back in another area, but first it's important to remember that this is not for the rest of your life. We just need you to rearrange some things for a little while until you're feeling better.

The patient who overestimates the *energy* an assignment requires benefits from similar questions. In the next example, the patient has a dysfunctional (and distorted) image of fulfilling an assignment.

T: What could get in the way of your going to the mall every day this week?

P: (*Sighs.*) I don't know if I'll have the energy.

T: What are you envisioning?

P: Well, I see me dragging myself into one store after another.

T: You know, we talked about your going just for 10 minutes every day. How many stores would you actually get to in 10 minutes? I wonder if you could be imagining that this assignment will be more difficult than we had planned?

In a different situation, the patient has correctly recalled the assignment but again overestimates the energy it will require. The therapist first helps *specify the problem* by doing a modified, short version of covert rehearsal.

P: I'm not sure I'll have the energy to take Max to the park for 15 minutes.

T: Will the problem be mostly getting out of the house, going to the park, or what you'll have to do *at* the park?

P: Getting out of the house. I have to get so much stuff together—his diaper bag, the stroller, a bottle, his coat and boots— [The therapist and patient then problem-solve; one solution is for her to gather all the necessities earlier in the day when she is feeling more energetic and less overwhelmed.]

In a third situation, the therapist simply sets up the assignment as an experiment.

P: I'm not sure I'll have the energy to make the phone calls.

T: Since we've run short of time today, how about if we just set up this assignment as an experiment: Let's write down your prediction, and next session, you can tell me how accurate it was. Is that okay?

Perfectionism

Many patients benefit from a simple reminder that they need not strive for perfection when doing homework:

T: Sally, learning to be assertive is a skill, like learning the computer. You'll get better with practice. So, if you have any trouble this week, don't worry. We'll figure out how to do it better at our next session.

Other patients with a strong underlying assumption about the necessity of being perfect may benefit from assignments that *include* mistakes:

T: It sounds as if your belief about perfectionism is showing up in difficulty doing therapy homework.

P: Yeah, it is.

T: How about this week if we have you do a Dysfunctional Thought Record which is *deliberately* imperfect? You could do it with messy handwriting or not do it thoroughly or don't look up correct spelling or put a 10-minute time limit on it or something like that.

Psychological Obstacles Masked as Practical Problems

Some patients propose that practical problems such as lack of time, energy, or opportunity may prevent them from carrying out an assignment. If the therapist believes that a thought or belief may also be interfering, he may investigate this possibility *before* discussing the practical problem.

T: Okay, so you're not sure if you'll be able to do this assignment [because of a practical problem]. Let's pretend for a moment that this problem magically disappears. How likely *now* are you do to the homework? Would anything else interfere? Any thoughts that would get in the way?

Problems Related to the Therapist's Cognitions

Finally, the therapist should assess whether any of *his* thoughts or beliefs hinder him from assertively and appropriately encouraging a patient to do homework. Typical dysfunctional assumptions of therapists include these:

"I'll hurt her feelings if I explore why she didn't do the homework."
"She'll get angry if I [nicely] confront her."
"She'll be insulted if I suggest she try a homework monitor."
"She doesn't really need to do homework to get better."
"She is too overburdened now with other things."
"She's too passive–aggressive to do homework."
"She's too fragile to expose herself to an anxious situation."

The therapist should ask himself what goes through *his* mind when he thinks about assigning homework or exploring why a patient has not done homework. Then a Dysfunctional Thought Record, a behavioral experiment, or a consultation with a supervisor or peer might be in order. He should remind himself that he is not doing his patient a favor if he allows her to skip homework and does not make extensive efforts to gain compliance.

REVIEWING HOMEWORK

It is important from the very beginning for patients to understand that homework is a vital part of therapy. The therapist therefore takes care always to attend to homework assigned at the previous session. Even if the patient is in crisis or wishes to discuss items unrelated to the homework, it is still useful to spend a few minutes discussing homework or to agree to discuss it at the next session.

Sometimes homework will be intimately connected with the agenda items and/or the therapist's goals and most of the session will involve homework items. Most of the time there will be some connection and homework review may take 5 to 15 minutes. A review of the homework may also lead to the assignment of new homework for the forthcoming week: to continue a task, for example, or to try a new task.

In summary, both therapist and patient should view homework as an essential part of therapy. Homework, properly assigned and completed, speeds up progress and allows the patient to practice the techniques of therapy which she will need when therapy is over.

Chapter 15

TERMINATION AND RELAPSE PREVENTION

The goal in cognitive therapy is to facilitate the remission of the patient's disorder and to teach the patient to be her own therapist, not for the therapist to solve all her problems. In fact, a therapist who views himself as responsible for helping the patient with *every* problem risks engendering or reinforcing dependence and deprives the patient of the opportunity to test and strengthen her skills. Therapy sessions are usually scheduled once a week initially. In an ideal situation, once the patient has experienced a reduction in symptoms and has learned basic cognitive therapy tools, therapy is gradually tapered, on a trial basis, to once every 2 weeks and then to once every 3 to 4 weeks. In addition, patients are encouraged to schedule "booster" sessions approximately 3, 6, and 12 months after termination. This chapter outlines steps to prepare the patient for termination and possible relapse from the start of therapy to the final booster session.

SESSION ONE ACTIVITIES

The therapist begins to prepare the patient for termination and relapse even in the first session. It is helpful to identify the patient's expectations for progress: how she expects to get better, how long she thinks it will take, whether she believes she should steadily make progress each week without setbacks. Patients benefit from a visual depiction of the course of progress, with periods of improvement which are typically interrupted (temporarily) by plateaus, fluctuations, or setbacks (see Figure 15.1).

If the therapist prepares the patient for fluctuations and setbacks from the very beginning, it is less likely that the patient will catastrophize

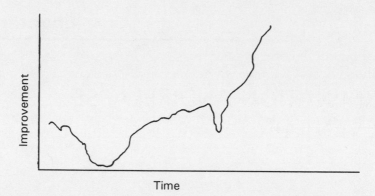

FIGURE 15.1. Progress in therapy. This graph, if skillfully drawn, can be made to resemble the southern border of the United States, with setbacks represented by "Texas" and "Florida." While striking some patients and therapists as humorous, this illustration may help patients recall that setbacks are normal.

if and when they occur. The therapist also stresses that life after therapy may be marked by occasional setbacks or difficulties but that the patient will be better equipped to handle them on her own.

THERAPIST: Many patients expect to get a little bit better every week. Is that what you think, too?

PATIENT: I really don't know.

T: Well, I'd like to take a minute to show you how you might progress so it won't bother you as much if you don't improve every single week.

P: Okay.

T: Now each patient is different, but very few actually make the same progress every week. Most patients have ups and downs. They go along, feeling a little better and a little better, then at some point, they reach a plateau or have a setback. Then they feel a little better and a little better, and then there may be another plateau or setback. So it's *normal* to have ups and downs. . . . Can you see why it's important to remember that in the future?

P: I guess so I won't worry so much about the down parts.

T: Exactly. You can remember back to this discussion where we predicted some low points. In fact, you might want to refer to a graph, which I'll draw for you now [Figure 15.1]. This is a rough idea of what might happen. Do you see that the setbacks get fewer and shorter and generally less severe as time goes on?

P: Uh huh.

T: Do you see if you were at the bottom of a setback that you'd be tempted to think you weren't getting better instead of seeing the whole picture?

P: Yeah.

T: These ups and downs may continue even after therapy. Of course, by then, you'll have the tools you need to help yourself. Or you may want to come in again for a session or two. We'll discuss this toward the end of therapy.

P: Okay.

T: Now, we don't know for sure just how you'll do in therapy. The important thing to remember is that it's normal to have ups and downs. And you'll be learning to be your own therapist so when therapy is over, you'll know how to deal with the downs yourself.

ACTIVITIES THROUGHOUT THERAPY

Attributing Progress to the Patient

The therapist is alert for opportunities to reinforce the patient for her progress. When a patient's mood has improved, the therapist ascertains the patient's attribution and reinforces the notion, whenever possible, that the patient has brought about changes in her thinking, mood, and/or behavior through her own efforts.

T: It sounds as if your depression is much lower this week. Why do you think that happened?

P: I'm not sure.

T: Did you do anything differently this week? Did you go ahead and do the activities we scheduled? Or did you respond to your negative thoughts?

P: Yeah. I actually exercised every day, and I went out with friends twice. A couple of times I caught myself criticizing myself, and I did a Dysfunctional Thought Record [DTR].

T: Is it possible you're feeling better this week because you did a number of things that helped?

P: Yes, I think so.

T: So what can you say about how you made progress?

P: I guess when I do things to help myself, I *do* feel better.

Some patients initially believe that all the credit for feeling better rightfully goes to the therapist. An alternative attribution—that the *patient* is responsible for positive changes—can fortify the patient's belief in her own self-efficacy (which is important to prevent relapse after therapy).

T: Why do you think you're feeling better this week?

P: You really helped me last session.

T: Well, I may have taught you *some* things, but who was it who actually changed around your thinking and your behavior this week?

P: It was me.

T: How much do you believe, then, that it's really *you* who deserves the credit?

Alternatively, the patient may attribute all the improvement to a change in circumstance (e.g., "I'm feeling better because my boyfriend called me") or to medication. The therapist acknowledges such factors but also asks about changes in the patient's thinking or behavior that could have contributed to or helped maintain her improvement.

If the patient persists in believing that she does not deserve credit, the therapist might decide to pursue her underlying belief ("What does it mean to you that I'm trying to give you credit?").

Teaching and Using Tools/Techniques Learned in Therapy

When teaching a patient techniques and tools, the therapist stresses that these are lifelong aids the patient can use in a number of situations now and in the future—that is, these techniques are not specific to just one disorder such as depression, but they can be used whenever the patient realizes she is reacting in an overly emotional or dysfunctional way. Common techniques and tools that can be used during and after therapy include the following:

1. Breaking down big problems into manageable components.
2. Generating alternative responses to problems.
3. Identifying, testing, and responding to automatic thoughts and beliefs.
4. Using Dysfunctional Thought Records.
5. Monitoring and scheduling activities.

6. Doing relaxation exercises.
7. Using distraction and refocusing techniques.
8. Creating and working one's way through hierarchies of difficult tasks.
9. Writing positive self-statement logs.
10. Identifying advantages and disadvantages (of specific thoughts, beliefs, behaviors, or choices when making a decision).

The therapist directly helps the patient see how she can use these tools in other situations during and after therapy:

T: Well, it seems as if identifying your depressing thoughts and then questioning and responding to them really reduced your sadness.

P: Yes, it did. I was surprised.

T: Did you know you could use these same tools whenever you feel you're overreacting—when you think you feel more anger, anxiety, sadness, embarrassment, than the situation calls for?

P: I hadn't really thought of it.

T: Now I'm not saying you should try to get rid of *all* negative emotion—only when you think you might be *over*reacting. Can you think of any other situations that came up in the last few weeks which you could have used a Dysfunctional Thought Record for?

P: (*Pauses.*) Nothing really comes to mind.

T: Any situations coming up in the next few weeks where it might be helpful to use a DTR?

P: (*Pauses.*) Well, I know I'm going to be really angry at my brother if he decides to stay at school for the summer instead of coming home.

T: What do you think of doing a DTR on this situation, writing down and then responding to your thoughts?

P: Sounds good.

Preparing for Setbacks during Therapy

As soon as the patient has begun to feel better, the therapist prepares her for a potential setback by asking her to imagine what will go through her mind if she starts to feel worse. Common responses include: "I shouldn't be feeling this way"; "This means I'm not getting better"; "I'm hopeless"; "I'll never get well"; "My therapist will be disappointed"; *or* "My therapist isn't doing a good job"; "Cognitive therapy doesn't work for me"; "I'm doomed to be depressed forever"; "It was only a fluke that

I felt better initially"; *or* the patient may report an image, for example, feeling frightened, alone, sad, huddled in the corner of her bed. The therapist helps the patient respond to these thoughts and images and to write a coping card. He may introduce or review the "progress in therapy" graph (Figure 15.1).

T: Well, you've really been making nice progress. Your depression seems to be lifting quite a bit.

P: I *am* feeling better.

T: Do you remember that we discussed setbacks at our first session?

P: A little.

T: Since it's possible you *could* have a setback, I'd like to discuss in advance how you could handle it.

P: Okay.

T: I'd like you to imagine for a moment that you've had a bad week. Nothing seems to have gone well. Everything looks black again. You're really down on yourself. It seems hopeless. Can you get a picture of that in your mind?

P: Yes. It's like it was before therapy.

T: Okay. Tell me what's going through your mind now.

P: (*Pauses.*) It's not fair. I was doing so well. This isn't working.

T: Good. Now, how can you answer these thoughts?

P: I'm not sure.

T: Well, you have a choice. You can continue to think these depressing thoughts. What do you predict will happen to your mood?

P: I'll probably feel worse.

T: *Or* you can remind yourself that this is only a setback, which is normal and temporary. Then how would you feel?

P: Better, probably, or at least not worse.

T: Okay. Having reminded yourself that setbacks are normal, what kinds of things have you learned to do in the past few weeks that could help you now?

P: I could do a DTR or get my mind off of it by concentrating on what I have to do.

T: Or both.

P: Right, or both.

T: Is there a reason to expect that the tools which helped you before won't help you again?

P: No.

T: So you can evaluate your negative thoughts, answer them back [hopefully on a DTR], and start concentrating on something else. Do you think it's worth writing down what we just talked about so you'll have a plan in case you do have a setback at some point?

NEAR TERMINATION ACTIVITIES

Responding to Concerns about Tapering Sessions

Several weeks before termination, the therapist discusses tapering sessions from once a week to once every other week or so as an experiment. Although some patients readily agree to this arrangement, others become anxious. It is useful for this latter group of patients to list verbally and perhaps record in writing the advantages of trying to reduce the frequency of visits. If a patient fails to see advantages, the therapist uses Socratic questions to help her see what these might be. They also discuss disadvantages so the therapist has an opportunity to help the patient reframe these disadvantages. (See Figure 15.2.)

The following transcript illustrates how such a discussion might proceed:

T: In our last session, we briefly discussed the possibility of experimenting with spacing our therapy sessions. Did you think about going to an every-other-week schedule on a trial basis?

P: I did. It made me a little anxious.

T: What went through your mind?

P: Oh, what if something happens that I can't deal with? What if I start getting more depressed—I couldn't stand that.

T: Did you evaluate these thoughts?

P: Yeah. I realized I was catastrophizing, that it wasn't the absolute end of therapy. And you did say I could call you if I needed to.

T: That's right. Did you imagine a specific situation that might come up that would be difficult?

P: No, not really.

T: Maybe it would help if we had you imagine a specific problem now.

P: Okay. [The patient imagines getting a low grade on a test, identifies

Advantages of tapering therapy

1. I'll have more opportunity to use and sharpen my tools.

2. I'll be less dependent on [my therapist].

3. I can use the therapy fee for other things.

4. I can spend more time [doing other things].

Disadvantages	Reframe
1. I might relapse.	If I'm going to relapse, it's better for it to happen while I'm still in therapy so I can learn how to handle it.
2. I may not be able to solve problems myself.	Tapering therapy gives me the chance to test my idea that I *need* [my therapist]. In the long run, it's better for me to learn to solve problems myself, because I won't be in therapy forever.
3. I'll miss [my therapist].	This is probably true but I *will* be able to tolerate it and it will encourage me to build up a support network.

FIGURE 15.2. Advantages and disadvantages (to Sally) of tapering therapy.

her automatic thoughts, responds to the thoughts, and makes a specific plan for what to do next.]

T: Now, let's talk about the second automatic thought you had about spacing our sessions—that you'd get more depressed and that you wouldn't be able to stand it.

P: I guess that may not be quite true. You've made me realize that I could stand to feel bad again. But I wouldn't like it.

T: Okay. Now let's say you *do* get more depressed and it's still a week and a half before our next session. What can you do?

P: Well, I can do what I did about a month ago. Reread my therapy notes, make sure I stay active, do more DTRs. Somewhere in my notes I have a list of things to do.

T: Would it be helpful to find that list now?

P: Yeah. It would help if I knew there was something I *could* do to feel better.

T: Okay. How about for homework if you find the list and write a DTR for these two thoughts: "Something might happen that I couldn't deal with," and "I couldn't stand it if I got more depressed."

P: Okay.

T: Any other thoughts about spacing our sessions?

P: Just that I'd miss not having you to talk to every week.

T: I'll miss that, too. Is there anyone else you could talk to, even a little?

P: Well, I could tell my roommate some things. And I guess I could call my brother.

T: That sounds like a good idea. Do you want to write that down to do, too?

P: Okay.

T: And finally, do you remember that we said we could *experiment* with every-other-week sessions? If it's not working well, we can always return to weekly sessions.

Responding to Concerns about Termination

When the patient is doing well with biweekly sessions, the therapist might suggest monthly sessions in preparation for termination. Again, tapering can be viewed as an experiment. At each succeeding session, the therapist and patient agree either to continue spacing sessions or to return to more frequent sessions.

As termination approaches, it is important to elicit the patient's automatic thoughts about termination. Some patients are excited and hopeful. At the other extreme, some patients are fearful or even angry. Most have some mixed feelings. They are pleased about their progress but concerned about relapse. Often they are sorry to end their relationship with the therapist.

It is important both to acknowledge the patient's feelings and to help her respond to any distortions. Often it is desirable for the therapist to express his own genuine feelings: some regret to the (gradual) ending of the relationship but pride in the patient's achievements through therapy and the hopeful expectation that the patient is ready to make it on her own. Responding to other automatic thoughts and examining advantages and disadvantages of termination can be carried out in the same way as was previously described in responding to thoughts about tapering sessions.

Reviewing What Was Learned in Therapy

The therapist encourages the patient to read through and organize all her therapy notes so she can easily refer to them in the future. For homework, she may write a synopsis of the important points and skills she learned in therapy and review this list with the therapist.

Self-Therapy Sessions

Although many patients do not follow through with formal self-therapy sessions, it is nevertheless useful to discuss a self-therapy plan (see Figure 15.3) and to encourage its use. The patient may try self-therapy sessions while regular therapy sessions are being tapered. In this way the patient can consult the therapist about problems in doing self-therapy (not enough time, misunderstandings about what to do) and about interfering thoughts (e.g., "This is too much work; I don't really need to do it; I can't do it on my own"). In addition to helping the patient respond to these problems, the therapist reminds the patient of the advantages of self-therapy sessions: The patient is continuing therapy but at her own convenience and without charge, she can keep her newly learned tools fresh and ready to use, she can resolve difficulties before they become major problems, she reduces the possibility of relapse; and she can use her skills to enrich her life in a variety of contexts.

A generic self-therapy plan is presented in Figure 15.3. The therapist reviews it with the patient and tailors it to meet her needs. Many patients benefit from a brief discussion of a reminder system: "Initially, you might want to try a self-therapy session once a week, then taper it to once or twice a month, then to once a season, and eventually, to once a year. How could you remind yourself to pull out this self-therapy plan periodically?"

Preparing for Setbacks after Termination

As mentioned previously, the therapist prepares the patient for setbacks early in treatment. Nearing termination, the therapist encourages the patient to compose a coping card specifying what to do if a setback occurs after therapy has ended. They can discuss such a card in session, and the patient can write the card in session or for homework. (See Figure 15.4 for a typical card.)

It is desirable for the patient to attempt to resolve her difficulties on her own before calling her therapist. She may indeed be able to handle the problems or setback on her own. If she is unsuccessful, at least she has had an opportunity to use her skills once more. If she does need another appointment, the therapist can help the patient discover what got in the way of her handling the setback or problem independently, and they can plan what the patient can do differently in the future.

GUIDE TO SELF-THERAPY SESSIONS

1. *Set agenda*
   - What important issues/situations should I think about?

2. *Review homework*
   - What did I learn?
   - If I didn't do homework, what got in the way (practical problems; automatic thoughts)?
   - What can I do to make it more likely I'll do homework this time?
   - What should I continue to do for homework?

3. *Review of past week(s)*
   - Other than a specific homework assignment, did I use any cognitive therapy tools?
   - Looking back, would it have been advantageous to have used cognitive therapy tools more?
   - How will I remember to use the tools next time?
   - What positive things happened during the week? What do I deserve credit for?
   - Did any problems come up? If so, how well did I handle them? If the problem recurred, how would I handle it next time?

4. *Think about current problematic issues/situations*
   - Am I viewing this realistically? Am I overreacting?
   - Is there another way of viewing this?
   - What should I do?

5. *Predict possible problems that may occur between now and the next therapy session*
   - What problems may come up in the next few days or weeks?
   - What should I do if the problem does arise?
   - Would it help to imagine myself coping with the problem?
   - What *positive* events do I have to look forward to?

6. *Set new homework*
   - What homework would be helpful? Should I consider:
     a. Doing DTRs
     b. Monitoring my activities
     c. Scheduling pleasure or mastery activities
     d. Working on a behavioral hierarchy
     e. Reading therapy notes
     f. Practicing skills such as relaxation or dealing with images
     g. Doing a positive self-statement log
   - Which behaviors would I like to change?

7. *Schedule the next self-therapy appointment*
   - When should the next appointment be? How much time should elapse?
   - Should I have future appointments on a regular basis: the first of each week/month/season?

FIGURE 15.3. Guide to self-therapy sessions. Copyright 1993 by Judith S. Beck, Ph.D.

What I can do in case of setback

1. I have a choice. I can catastrophize about the setback, get myself all upset, think things are hopeless, and probably feel worse. Or I can look back over my therapy notes, remember that setbacks are a normal part of recovery, and see what I can learn from this setback. Doing these things will probably make me feel better and make the setback less severe.

2. Next, I should have a self-therapy session and plan how to resolve my current difficulties.

3. Third, I can call [my therapist] and briefly tell him about the work I've done on my own and/or discuss [with him] the possibility of another regular therapy session if it seems to be in my best interest.

FIGURE 15.4. Sally's coping card about setbacks.

BOOSTER SESSIONS

The therapist encourages the patient to schedule booster sessions after termination for several reasons. If any difficulties have arisen, the patient and therapist can discuss how the patient handled them and assess whether she could have handled them in a better way. Together patient and therapist can look ahead to the next several weeks and months and predict future difficulties that could arise. They then formulate a plan to deal with these situations. Knowing that the therapist will ask about her progress doing self-therapy may motivate the patient to do her cognitive therapy homework and practice her skills. In addition, the therapist can help the patient determine whether her previously modified dysfunctional beliefs have been reactivated. If so, they can do cognitive restructuring in session and plan for continued belief work at home.

Booster sessions also afford the therapist an opportunity to check on the reemergence of dysfunctional strategies (such as avoidance). The patient can express any new or previously unaccomplished goals and develop a plan to work toward them. Together the therapist and patient can evaluate the self-therapy program and modify as needed. Finally, knowing she is scheduled for booster sessions after termination sometimes allays the patient's anxiety about maintaining her progress on her own.

In order to prepare for booster sessions, the therapist may provide the patient with a list of questions (see Figure 15.5).

As the following transcript indicates, the therapist's overall goal for

GUIDE TO BOOSTER SESSIONS

A. Schedule ahead—make definite appointments, if possible, and call to confirm.

B. Consider coming as a preventive measure, even if you have been maintaining your progress.

C. Prepare before you come. Decide what would be helpful to discuss, including:

    1. What has gone well for you?

    2. What problems arose? How did you handle them? Was there a better way of handling them?

    3. What problem(s) could arise between this booster session and your next booster session? Imagine the problem in detail. What automatic thoughts might you have? What beliefs might be activated? How will you deal with the automatic thoughts/beliefs? How will you problem-solve?

    4. What cognitive therapy work did you do? What cognitive therapy work would you like to do between now and the next booster session? What automatic thoughts might get in the way of doing the cognitive therapy work? How will you answer these thoughts?

    5. What further goals do you have for yourself? How will you achieve them? How can the things you learned in cognitive therapy help?

FIGURE 15.5. Guide to booster sessions. Copyright 1993 by Judith S. Beck, Ph.D.

the booster session is to check on the patient's well-being and plan for continued maintenance or progress.

T: I'm glad you were able to come in today. It looks from the Depression Inventory that you're a little more depressed than at termination?

P: Yes, I just recently broke up with my boyfriend.

T: I'm sorry to hear that. Do you think that situation accounted for the entire rise in your score?

P: I think so. I was feeling pretty good until last week.

T: Is the breakup something you'd like to put on the agenda to talk about today?

P: Yes, that and my progress, or rather lack of progress, in looking for a summer job.

T: Okay. And I'd like to find out how things have been going for you generally, aside from the breakup. Whether you encountered any other rough spots and how you dealt with them, how much cognitive therapy homework you were able to do, any difficulties you think may arise in the next 2 or 3 months.

P: Okay.

T: Would you like to start with the breakup? Can you tell me how it came about? [They briefly discuss the breakup. The therapist is concerned with how the patient reacted to the breakup, whether old dysfunctional beliefs have been activated.] (*Summarizing.*) So things had begun to deteriorate, and he told you he wanted to start seeing other women? When he told you that, what went through your mind?

P: That he didn't really love me.

T: And what did that mean to you, that he didn't love you?

P: It meant that I'd have to find somebody else.

T: And what did that mean to you, that you'd have to find somebody else?

P: Well, it'll be hard.

T: And what does that mean to you, that it'll be hard?

P: I guess it means I'm not very lovable.

T: How much did you believe that you weren't very lovable right when he told you he wanted to see other women?

P: Oh, about 90%

T: And how much do you believe it now?

P: Less, maybe 50%, 60%.

T: What made the difference?

P: Well, part of me knows that we probably just weren't right for each other.

T: So you were able to modify this old idea of not being lovable.

P: Somewhat.

T: Right. Now what did you learn from therapy that you can do to damp down this unlovable idea further and strengthen the idea that you are lovable?

P: I probably should do a DTR on it. And I know my therapy notes have a lot on it. I should have gone back and reread them.

T: That might have helped. Did you think of doing that?

P: Yeah. I guess I thought it really wouldn't help.

T: What do you think now?

P: Well, it helped me before, it should help me again.

T: What would get in the way of going home and doing some work on it in the next couple of days?

P: Nothing. I'll do it. I think it probably will help.

T: Now might this thought, "It won't help," pop up again the next time you're going through a rough spot?

P: It might.

T: What could you do now so it would be more likely that you'd test that thought?

P: What could I do *now*?

T: Yeah. What could you do to remind yourself that you had the thought *this* time and then realized it might not be true?

P: I should write it down, maybe on a paper I keep in my desk.

T: Okay, how about if you write down some of the things we just talked about—doing a DTR on being unlovable, reading through your therapy notes, writing a response to the thought, "It won't help," to put in your desk.

In this portion of the booster session, the therapist assesses the patient's level of depression, sets the agenda, discusses one issue, and helps the patient set homework for herself. The therapist ascertains that the patient is very mildly depressed and the elevation seems related only to the breakup of the relationship. (Had the depression been more severe, the therapist would have spent more time assessing triggers and identifying and modifying dysfunctional beliefs, thoughts, and behaviors. The therapist and patient might have discussed the advisability of an additional session or sessions.)

This patient is easily able to express her automatic thought and underlying belief. She and the therapist spend little time developing a plan to help her modify her ideas; she had already learned the tools during therapy. She needed the booster session to remind her to use the tools.

In summary, relapse prevention is carried on throughout therapy. Problems in tapering sessions and in termination are addressed as any other problems, with a combination of problem-solving and responding to dysfunctional thoughts and beliefs.

Chapter 16

TREATMENT PLANNING

A t any given moment in therapy, how does the therapist decide what to say or do next? Partial answers to this question have been provided throughout this book, but this chapter provides a more coherent framework for making decisions and planning treatment. To keep the therapy focused and moving in the right direction, the therapist continually asks himself, "What is the specific problem here and what am I trying to accomplish?" He is cognizant of his objectives in the current portion of the session, in the session as a whole, in the current stage of therapy, and in therapy as a whole. This chapter outlines a number of areas essential to effective treatment planning: accomplishing broad therapeutic goals, planning treatment across sessions, devising treatment plans, planning individual sessions, deciding whether to focus on a problem, and modifying standard treatment for specific disorders.

ACCOMPLISHING BROAD THERAPEUTIC GOALS

At the broadest level, the therapist wishes to facilitate a remission of the patient's disorder and prevent relapse. To do so, he aims not only to reduce the patient's symptoms by helping her to modify her dysfunctional thoughts, beliefs, and behaviors but also to teach and motivate her to continue such modification on her own after termination—in other words, to continue to be her own therapist. In order to accomplish these broad goals, the therapist does the following:

1. Builds a sound therapeutic alliance with the patient.
2. Makes explicit the structure and the process of therapy to the patient.

3. Teaches the patient the cognitive model and shares his conceptualization of the patient with her.
4. Helps alleviate the patient's distress through cognitive and behavioral techniques and problem-solving.
5. Teaches the patient how to use these techniques herself, helps her generalize the use of the techniques, and motivates her to use the techniques in the future.

PLANNING TREATMENT ACROSS SESSIONS

The therapist develops a general plan for therapy and a specific plan for each individual session. Therapy can be viewed in three phases: beginning, middle, and end. In the beginning phase of treatment (see Chapter 4), the therapist plans to accomplish a number of goals: build a strong therapeutic alliance; identify and specify the patient's goals for therapy; solve problems; teach the patient the cognitive model; get the patient behaviorally activated (particularly if she is depressed and withdrawn); educate the patient about her disorder; teach the patient to identify, evaluate, and respond to her automatic thoughts; socialize the patient (into doing homework, setting an agenda in therapy, and providing feedback to the therapist); and instruct the patient in coping strategies. In the first phase of therapy, the therapist often takes the lead in suggesting agenda items and homework assignments.

In the middle phase of therapy, the therapist continues working toward the above objectives but also emphasizes on identifying, evaluating, and modifying the patient's beliefs. He shares his cognitive conceptualization of the patient with her and uses both "rational" and "emotional" techniques to facilitate belief modification. In addition, the therapist (when applicable) helps the patient to reformulate her goals and teaches her skills she lacks but needs to accomplish her goals.

In the final phase of therapy, the emphasis shifts to preparing for termination and preventing relapse (see Chapter 15). By this point, the patient has become much more active in therapy, taking the lead in setting the agenda, suggesting solutions to problems, and devising homework assignments.

DEVISING A TREATMENT PLAN

The therapist develops a treatment plan based on the patient's evaluation, her Axis I and Axis II symptoms and disorder(s), and her specific presenting problems. Sally, for example, set four goals in the first therapy session: to improve her school work, to decrease her anxiety about tests, to meet more people, and to join some school activities. Based on her intake evaluation and these goals, her therapist devised a general therapy plan (see Figure 16.1). In each individual session, he works on several of the areas specified in the plan based on what they covered in the previous session(s), what Sally has done for homework, and what problems or topics Sally puts on the agenda that day. The therapist also takes each individual problem or goal and does a critical analysis, either mentally or on paper (see Figure 16.2).

Having formulated a general treatment plan, the therapist adheres to it to a greater or lesser degree, revising it as necessary. Analyzing specific problems compels him to conceptualize the patient's difficulties in detail and to formulate a treatment plan tailored for her. Doing so also helps him focus each individual session, grasp the flow of therapy from one session to the next, and become more cognizant of progress.

PLANNING INDIVIDUAL SESSIONS

Before and during a session, the therapist asks himself a number of questions to formulate an overall plan for the session and to guide him as he conducts the therapy session. At the most general level, he asks himself, "What am I trying to accomplish, and how can I do so most efficiently?" The experienced therapist automatically reflects on many specific issues. The following list of questions, while potentially daunting to the beginner, is a useful guide for more advanced therapists who wish to improve their ability to make better decisions about how to proceed within a therapy session. The list is designed to be read and considered before a therapy session as conscious contemplation of the questions during a session would undoubtedly interfere with the therapeutic process.

1. As the therapist reviews his notes from the previous session *before the session*, he asks himself:

SALLY'S TREATMENT PLAN

1. Problem-solve how to improve her concentration, seek needed help in her courses, meet more people, and join activities.
2. Help her identify, evaluate, and respond to automatic thoughts about herself, school, other people, and therapy, especially those that are particularly distressing and/or hinder her from solving problems.
3. Investigate dysfunctional beliefs about perfectionism and seeking help from others.
4. Discuss her self-criticism and increase giving herself credit.
5. Decrease the amount of time she spends in bed.

FIGURE 16.1. Sally's treatment plan.

PROBLEM ANALYSIS

A. Typical problem situations

Situation	→ Automatic thoughts	→	Emotions, behavior, physiological reaction
Sitting in library	→ I'll never get this done. I don't understand. I'll never understand this. I'm so stupid. I'll probably flunk out.	→ Sad → Stops studying	→ (Not applicable)
Studying in room at night	→ This is hopeless.	→ Sad → Lies on bed	→ Cries

B. Dysfunctional behaviors:

Keeps going over and over some material when comprehension is poor or stops studying altogether.
Fails to respond to automatic thoughts.
Doesn't ask others for help.

C. Cognitive distortions:

Attributes problem to weakness in self rather than to depression.
Assumes future is hopeless.
Assumes she is helpless and can't do anything about the problem.
Possibly equates her worth with her achievement?

D. Therapeutic strategies:

1. Do problem-solving. Switch to another subject if comprehension is low after a second reading. Devise a plan to get formal or informal help from professors, teaching assistant, tutor, or classmate. Compose coping cards in session to be read before and during studying.
2. Monitor moods. Use activity monitor to mark study periods and rate (0–10) the severity of anxiety and/or sadness. When anxiety or sadness is greater than 3, jot down the automatic thoughts.
3. Use Socratic questioning to evaluate automatic thoughts. Teach use of Dysfunctional Thought Record.
4. Use guided discovery to uncover meaning of automatic thoughts; put in conditional (If . . . then . . .) format and test.
5. If applicable, use cognitive continuum to illustrate that achievement is on a continuum, rather than consisting of either perfection or failure.

FIGURE 16.2. Analysis of problem 1: Difficulty studying.

a. What is the patient's disorder(s)? How severe is it now compared to the beginning of therapy?
b. How, if at all, does standard cognitive therapy need to be varied for treatment of this disorder and this patient in particular?

    c. How have I conceptualized the patient's difficulties? (Therapist may refer to a Cognitive Conceptualization Diagram.)

    d. At which stage (beginning, middle, final) of therapy is the patient? How many sessions do we have left (if there is a limit)?

    e. What are the patient's major problems and goals? How much progress have we made on each one so far? Which one(s) have we been focusing on recently?

    f. What progress has been made so far in the patient's mood, behavior, symptoms?

    g. How strong is our therapeutic alliance? What, if anything, do I need to do today to strengthen it?

    h. At which *cognitive* level have we primarily been working: automatic thought, intermediate belief, core belief, or a mixture? How much progress have we made at each level?

    i. What behavioral changes have we been working toward? How much progress have we made?

    j. What happened in the last few therapy sessions? What dysfunctional ideas or problems (if any) have hindered therapy? How do I want to handle them? What skills have we been working on? Which one(s) do I want to reinforce? Which new skills do I want to teach?

    k. What happened in the last session? What homework did the patient agree to do? What, if anything, did I agree to do (e.g., call her physician or recommend a book or article related to her difficulties)?

2. As the therapist begins the therapy session and checks on the *patient's mood*, he asks himself:

    a. How is she feeling compared to last session? Compared to the general course so far? Has she been making progress?

    b. Which mood predominates (e.g., sadness, anxiety, anger, or shame)?

    c. Do her objective scores match her subjective description? If not, why not?

    d. Is there anything about her mood we should put on the agenda to discuss more fully?

3. As the patient provides a *brief review of her week*, the therapist asks himself:

    a. How did this week go compared to previous weeks?

    b. What signs of progress are there?

    c. What problems came up this week?

    d. Did anything happen to make her more or less hopeful about therapy and about reaching her goals?

   e. Is there anything that happened this week that we should put
       on the agenda to discuss more fully?

4. As the therapist checks on the patient's *use of alcohol, drugs, and
medication* (if applicable), he asks himself:

   a. Is there a problem in any of these areas?
   b. Should we put any of these things on the agenda to discuss
       more fully?

5. As the therapist asks the patient about feedback from and highlights of the *previous session*, he asks himself:

   a. Does the patient seem to be honestly expressing her feed-
       back? If not, should I gently question her about it now? Put it
       on the agenda? Bring it up at another session?
   b. What do I need to do (if anything) to strengthen our thera-
       peutic alliance?
   c. Does the patient remember much about the last session? Can
       she express the most important points? If not, did she take
       adequate notes at the last session? Should I put this problem
       on the agenda?

6. As the therapist and patient *set the agenda*, the therapist asks
himself:

   a. Which problem looks like the most productive one to discuss?
       Which is most important to the patient? Which is the most
       resolvable? Which one is likely to bring about symptom relief
       within today's session?
   b. Which problem might be used to teach or reinforce a needed
       skill?
   c. Might it be *counterproductive* to discuss any item—for example,
       in an early session, is a particular problem too complex to
       resolve? Is a particular problem likely to activate a core belief
       more strongly when the patient does not yet have the tools to
       respond to the belief effectively?

7. As the therapist and patient *prioritize agenda items*, the therapist
asks himself:

   a. How much time will each agenda item take? How many items
       can we discuss?
   b. Are there any problems the patient could resolve herself,
       resolve with someone else, or bring up at another session?
   c. What is my major objective for the session: improvement in
       mood; cognitive change; problem-solving; behavioral
       change; improving the therapeutic alliance? Discussion of

which problems/items is most likely to accomplish this objective?

d. How do these problems/items mesh with what is most important to the patient?

e. How much time should we allot to each chosen item/problem?

8. As the therapist and patient *review the homework*, the therapist asks himself:

a. How is today's homework related to the agenda items? Should discussion of any of the homework tasks be postponed until we get to a specific agenda item?

b. How much of the homework did the patient do? If little, what got in the way?

c. Was the homework useful? If not, why not? If so, what did the patient learn?

d. How should we modify this week's homework to make it more effective?

9. As the therapist and patient discuss the *first agenda item*, the therapist asks himself questions in four areas:

Defining the Problem
a. What is the specific problem?
b. What are the specific situations in which the problem arises?
c. Why does the *patient* believe she has this problem? Why do *I* think the patient has this problem?
d. How does this problem fit into the overall cognitive conceptualization of the patient? How does it relate to her overall goals?
e. What role, if any, does the patient's thinking and behavior play in this problem?

Devising a Strategy
a. Can we do outright problem-solving? What thoughts and beliefs might interfere with problem-solving or carrying out a solution?
b. Which thought or belief should we work on to bring about needed behavioral change? What type of new but thematically related thought or belief would be more adaptive for this patient? How does this new thought or belief relate to the conceptualization?
c. What behavioral change can I suggest that might bring about needed cognitive change?

Choosing Techniques
a. What specifically am I trying to accomplish as we discuss this agenda item?
b. Which techniques have worked well for this patient (or for similar patients) in the past? Which techniques have *not* worked well?
c. Which technique should I try first?
d. How will I evaluate its effectiveness?
e. Will I employ the technique or employ it *and* teach it to the patient?

Monitoring the Process
a. Are we working together as a team?
b. Is the patient "buying" what I am leading her toward?
c. Is she having interfering automatic thoughts about herself, this technique, our therapy, me, the future?
d. Is her mood lifting?
e. How well is this technique working? Should we continue this technique? Should I try something else?
f. Will we finish discussion of this agenda item in time? If not, do I need to interrupt us and should we collaboratively decide to continue this item and curtail or eliminate discussion of another item?
g. What follow-up (*i.e.*, homework assignment) should I suggest to strengthen the patient's learning?
h. How will the patient remember the important things we are talking about? Is she taking adequate notes?

10. *Following discussion of the first agenda item,* the therapist asks himself:

a. How is the patient feeling now?
b. Do I need to do anything to reestablish rapport?
c. Did I arrange for follow-up to this item (e.g., a homework assignment, agreement to put the item on the agenda at our next session, or agreement to put off further discussion of it to a later date)?
d. How much time is left in the session? Do we have time for another agenda item? What should we do next?

11. *Before closing the session,* the therapist asks himself:

a. Do I need to probe further for negative feedback?
b. If there was negative feedback, how should I address it?
c. Did the patient understand the main thrust of the session?

      d. Will she remember whatever learning/skills I imparted? Did we set relevant homework assignments?

12. *After the session*, the therapist asks himself:

      a. How should I refine my conceptualization?

      b. What do I want to remember to address in the next session? Future sessions?

      c. Do I need to attend to our relationship?

      d. If I could do the session over again, what would I do differently?

DECIDING WHETHER TO FOCUS ON A PROBLEM

A critical decision in every therapy session is which problem (or problems) to pursue. Although the therapist collaborates in making this decision with the patient, he nevertheless guides therapy toward discussion of problems that are distressing, recurrent, and ongoing and toward which he judges they will be able to make some progress during the session. The therapist tends to limit discussion of problems that he judges the patient can solve herself, which are isolated incidents unlikely to recur, which are not particularly distressing, and/or which seem likely to lead to an unproductive use of therapy time.

    Having identified and specified a problem, the therapist does several things to help him decide how much time and effort to spend on the problem. He gathers more data about the problem, reviews his options, reflects on practical considerations, uses the stage of therapy as a guide, and changes the focus when necessary. These five steps are described below.

Gathering More Data about a Problem

When a patient first brings up a problem or when the existence of a problem becomes apparent in the midst of a session, the therapist assesses the nature of the problem to determine whether it seems worthwhile to intervene. For example, Sally has put a new problem on the agenda: Her father's business is failing, and Sally feels sad. The therapist questions her to assess how useful it will be to devote a significant portion of therapy time to this problem.

THERAPIST: Okay, you said you wanted to bring up something about your dad and his business?

PATIENT: Yeah. His business has been pretty rocky for a while, but now it looks as if it may go bankrupt.

T: (*Gathering more information.*) If it does go bankrupt, how will that affect you?

P: Oh, nothing directly. I just feel so bad for him. I mean, he'll still have enough money but . . . he's worked really hard for this.

T: (*Trying to discover whether there is a distortion in the patient's thinking.*) What do you think will happen if it does go bankrupt?

P: Well, he's already started looking for a new business. He's not the type to just lie around or take time off.

T: (*Still assessing whether the patient is thinking dysfunctionally.*) What's the worst part of this to you?

P: Just that he probably feels bad.

T: How do *you* feel when you think about his feeling badly?

P: Bad . . . sad.

T: How sad?

P: 75%

T: (*Testing whether the patient can take a long view.*) Do you have a sense that though he may feel badly initially, he won't stay that way indefinitely? That he'll probably get involved in another business and feel better?

P: Yeah, I think that'll probably happen.

T: Do you think you're feeling "normal" sadness over this? Or do you think this is affecting you *too* strongly?

P: I think I'm having a normal reaction.

T: (*Having assessed no further work on this problem is warranted.*) Anything else on this?

P: No, I don't think so.

T: Okay. I'm sorry this happened to your dad. Let me know what happens.

P: I will.

T: Should we turn to the next item on our agenda?

In another situation, the therapist determines that a problem *does* require intervention.

T: You wanted to talk about living arrangements for next year?

P: Yes. I'm pretty upset. My roommate and I have decided to live together again. She wants to live off campus. So we have to look for an apartment in West Philly or downtown. But she's going home for spring vacation so it's mostly up to me to find a place.

T: When were you feeling the most upset about this?

[Hypothesizing that the patient's distress is probably due to not knowing what to do, to anger at the roommate for leaving the work up to her, or to both, the therapist questions the patient specifically to uncover her automatic thoughts and emotions.]

P: Yesterday, when I agreed to start looking while she was away. . . . Actually, it was last night when I realized I didn't know what to do.

T: How were you feeling?

P: Overwhelmed . . . anxious.

T: What was going through your mind last night as you were thinking about this?

P: I don't know what to do. I don't even know where to start.

T: (*Seeking a fuller picture; determining whether there were other important automatic thoughts.*) What else was going through your mind?

P: I was asking myself, "What should I do first? I've never done this before. Should I go to a real estate agent? Should I look in *The Daily Pennsylvanian* [newspaper]?"

T: (*Still seeing whether there are any other important thoughts.*) Were you having any thoughts about your roommate?

P: No, not really. She said she'd help when she got back. She said I didn't have to start looking 'til then.

T: Were you making any predictions?

P: I don't know.

T: (*Giving an opposite example.*) Well, were you thinking you'd easily find a great place with a cheap rent?

P: No . . . no, I was thinking, "What if I find a place and it turns out to be infested with cockroaches, or unsafe, or too noisy, or in really bad shape?"

T: Did you have an image like that in your mind?

P: Yeah. Dark, smelly, dirty. (*Shudders.*)

Reviewing the Options

Now that the therapist has a fuller picture, he mentally reviews his options. He could do one or more of the following:

1. Engage Sally in straightforward problem-solving, helping her decide which steps seem the most reasonable and feasible.
2. Teach Sally problem-solving skills, using this problem as an example.
3. Use this situation as an opportunity to reinforce the cognitive model.
4. Use this situation as an opportunity to help Sally conceptualize her larger difficulty of *assuming* she is inadequate in a new situation and feeling overwhelmed instead of testing this belief.
5. Have Sally identify the most distressing thought and help her evaluate it.
6. Teach Sally how to do a Dysfunctional Thought Record using this situation.
7. Use the image she described as an opportunity to teach her imagery techniques.
8. Make a collaborative decision with Sally to move on to the next agenda item (perhaps to an even more pressing problem) and to return to this problem later in the session or in a future session.

Reflecting on Practical Considerations

How does the therapist decide which course to pursue? He takes into account a number of factors, including:

1. What is likely to bring Sally substantial relief?
2. What do they have time to do? What *else* do they need to do in the session?
3. What skills would be valuable to teach or review with Sally for which this problem provides an opportunity?
4. What, if anything, could Sally do herself (i.e., for homework) to relieve her distress? For example, if Sally is at the point where she could do a Dysfunctional Thought Record on this at home and feel better, they can spend session time on other things that will help her progress faster.

Using the Stage of Therapy as a Guide

The therapist is often guided by the patient's stage of therapy. For example, a therapist tends to avoid tackling a very distressing complex problem in the first few sessions with depressed patients if it is unlikely that they will make much headway toward it. He also tends to avoid discussing issues that activate a painful core belief early in therapy before the patient has the tools to deal with it.

Initial sessions are much more focused on solving *easier* problems, just as they are more focused on helping patients evaluate "easier" automatic thoughts rather than their more rigid, less malleable beliefs. Experiencing success in early sessions engenders hope in patients and makes them more motivated to work in therapy.

CHANGING THE FOCUS IN A SESSION

Sometimes the therapist can't easily assess how difficult a problem will be or how likely it is that a particular discussion will activate a painful core belief. In these cases, he may *initially* focus on a problem but switch to another topic when he realizes his interventions are not successful and/or the patient is experiencing greater (unintended) distress. Following is a transcript from an early therapy session.

T: Okay, next on the agenda. You said you'd like to meet more people. [They discuss this goal more specifically.] Now how could you meet new people this week?

P: . . . (*In a meek voice.*) I could talk to people at work.

T: (*Noticing that the patient suddenly looks downcast.*) What's going through your mind right now?

P: It's hopeless. I'll never be able to do it. I've tried this before. (*Appears angry.*) All my other therapists have tried this, too. But, I'm telling you, I just can't do it! It won't work!

The therapist hypothesizes from the patient's sudden negative affective shift that a core belief has been activated. He realizes that continuing in the same vein at this time will likely be counterproductive. Instead of refocusing on the problem, he decides to repair the therapeutic alliance by eliciting and then testing the patient's automatic thoughts about him (e.g., "When I asked you how you could meet more people this week, what thoughts did you have about *me*?"). Later he gives the patient a choice about whether or not to return to this agenda item (e.g., "I'm glad you can see that I hadn't intended to make you do things you're not ready for. Now, would you like to return to the topic of meeting new people or should we come back to it another time [at another session] and move on to the problem you had with your friend, Elise, this week?").

In summary, early in therapy the therapist tends to guide discussion *away* from the following:

1. A problem that is too complex (i.e., one in which substantial progress within the session is unlikely). An example of this is a long-standing marital conflict.

2. A problem that is too tightly tied to a very strong, very rigid belief (e.g., "If I am not 100% compliant with others' wishes, God will punish me").
3. A problem that is likely to activate a very painful core belief for which the patient lacks adequate coping tools (e.g., "I will be abandoned").
4. A problem that the patient can resolve on her own. If the therapist focuses on this type of problem, he is not making the most efficient use of therapy time.
5. A problem that the patient does not want to work on.
6. A problem that is not particularly distressing to the patient.

Difficult problems are not avoided but instead are tackled *after* a patient is feeling somewhat better and has learned more skills for dealing with the problem and the associated dysfunctional thoughts and beliefs.

MODIFYING STANDARD TREATMENT FOR SPECIFIC DISORDERS

It is essential for the therapist to have a solid understanding of the patient's current symptoms and functioning, presenting problems, precipitating events, and history before starting therapy. Equally important is a five-axis diagnosis according to DSM-IV. This book has discussed standard cognitive therapy for depression with associated anxiety. The following are brief descriptions of how the emphasis of therapy should be varied for other disorders. The therapist is urged to consult specialized texts (see below) for patients whose primary disorder is not a simple, unipolar depression.

1. *Panic disorder.* Therapy emphasizes the evaluation and testing of the patient's catastrophic misinterpretation that a specific benign symptom (or small set of symptoms) means that a specific physical or mental catastrophe is happening or is about to happen (Beck, 1987; Clark, 1989).

2. *Generalized anxiety disorder.* Therapy emphasizes teaching a patient to assess more realistically the threat of danger across situations and to assess and fortify her capacity to cope with threatening situations (Beck & Emery, 1985; Butler et al., 1991; Clark, 1989).

3. *Social phobias.* Therapy emphasizes cognitive restructuring, anxiety management techniques, and guided exposure. (Beck & Emery, 1985; Butler, 1989; Heimberg, 1990).

4. *Obsessive–compulsive disorder.* Therapy emphasizes exposure and response prevention and guiding the patient to discover experimentally

that her problem is her thoughts rather than the possible occurrence of a real-world problem (which she is trying to prevent through neutralizing behavior and attempts at controlling her thoughts). Among other things, the therapist helps the patient evaluate the degree to which she would realistically be responsible if an adverse circumstance happened to another person or to herself (Salkovskis & Kirk, 1989).

5. *Posttraumatic stress disorder.* Along with teaching patients techniques to manage their intense anxiety symptoms and recurrent distressing images, therapy emphasizes the identification and modification of the meaning the patient has attached to a traumatic event (Dancu & Foa, 1992; Parrott & Howes, 1991).

6. *Eating disorders.* Therapy emphasizes restructuring of dysfunctional beliefs about food, weight, and one's self (particularly in regard to body image and self-worth) (Bowers, 1993; Fairburn & Cooper, 1989; Garner & Bemis, 1985).

7. *Substance abuse.* Therapy emphasizes identifying and testing thoughts and images about taking drugs, modifying beliefs that increase risk of drug use, coping with drug cravings, and providing relapse prevention (Beck et al., 1993; Marlatt & Gordon, 1985).

8. *Personality disorders.* Therapy emphasizes improving current functioning (through increasing the patient's repertoire of compensatory strategies), developing and learning from the therapeutic relationship, understanding the historical development and maintenance of core beliefs and modifying core beliefs through both "rational" and experiential methods (Beck et al., 1990; Layden et al., 1993; Young, 1990).

9. *Schizophrenia.* As an adjunctive treatment in combination with pharmacotherapy, therapy emphasizes the consideration of alternative explanations for various psychotic experiences (Chadwick & Lowe, 1990; Kingdon & Turkington, 1994; Perris et al., 1993).

10. *Couples' problems.* Therapy emphasizes the individual's taking responsibility for modifying his/her dysfunctional expectations, beliefs, interpretations of, and behavior toward his/her partner (Baucom & Epstein, 1990; Beck, 1988; Dattilio & Padesky, 1990).

11. *Bipolar disorder.* As an adjunctive treatment, therapy emphasizes early identification of hypomanic and depressive episodes; strategies for dealing with these episodes; regularizing the patient's sleeping, eating, and activity levels; reducing the patient's vulnerability and exposure to triggering situations; and enhancing medication compliance (Palmer, Williams, & Adams, 1994).

These brief descriptions are intended to encourage the reader to seek additional training (whether formalized or self-instructed) for more complex disorders which require a variation of standard cognitive therapy.

In summary, effective treatment planning requires a sound diagnosis, a solid formulation of the case in cognitive terms, and consideration of the individual patient's characteristics and problems. Treatment is tailored to the individual; the therapist develops an overall strategy as well as a specific plan for each session, considering the following:

1. The patient's diagnosis(es).
2. A conceptualization of her difficulties (which he checks out with the patient for accuracy).
3. The patient's goals for therapy.
4. The patient's most pressing concerns.
5. The therapist's goals for therapy.
6. The stage of therapy.
7. The individual learning characteristics of the patient.
8. The motivation of the patient.
9. The nature and strength of the therapeutic alliance.

The therapist develops and continually modifies a general plan for treatment across sessions and a more specific plan before each session and within each session.

Chapter 17

PROBLEMS IN THERAPY

Problems of one kind or another arise with nearly every patient in cognitive therapy. Even experienced therapists who have mastered techniques encounter difficulties at times in establishing a therapeutic alliance, correctly conceptualizing a patient's difficulties, and consistently working toward joint objectives. A reasonable goal for a therapist is therefore not to avoid problems altogether but rather to learn to uncover and specify problems, to conceptualize how they arose, and to plan how to remediate them.

It is useful to view problems or stuck points in therapy as opportunities for the therapist to refine his conceptualization of the patient. In addition, problems in therapy often provide insight into problems the patient experiences outside the office. Finally, difficulties with one patient provide an opportunity for the therapist to refine his own skills, to promote his flexibility and creativity, and to gain new understandings and expertise in helping other patients, as problems can arise not just because of the patient's characteristics but also because of the therapist's relative weaknesses. This chapter describes how to uncover the existence of problems and how to conceptualize and remediate problems at stuck points in therapy.

UNCOVERING THE EXISTENCE OF A PROBLEM

The therapist uncovers the existence of a problem in a number of ways:

1. By listening to the patient's unsolicited feedback.
2. By directly soliciting the patient's feedback, whether or not she has provided verbal or nonverbal signals of a problem.
3. By reviewing audio- or videotapes of therapy sessions alone or with a colleague or supervisor.

4. By tracking progress according to objective tests and the
    patient's subjective report of symptom relief.

The easiest way to recognize that a problem has arisen in therapy is obviously when the patient states the problem directly (e.g., "Dr. Doe, I don't think you understand what I'm saying," or "I understand what you're saying *intellectually* but not in my gut"). Many patients, however, allude *indirectly* to a problem (e.g., "I see what you're saying, but I don't know if I could do it any other way," or, "I'll try," [implying that she believes she'll be unsuccessful in carrying out a task]). In these cases, the therapist questions the patient further to ascertain whether a problem does indeed exist and to determine the dimensions of the problem.

Many times, however, the patient fails to relate, either directly or indirectly, a problem with therapy. The therapist can uncover problems by adhering to the standard structure of the session (which includes asking the patient for feedback at the end of the session), by periodically checking on the depth of the patient's understanding during the session, and by eliciting the patient's automatic thoughts when he notices an affect shift during the session.

For example, on one occasion Sally's therapist sensed through nonverbal cues (a faraway look in her eyes, restless shifting in her seat) that she was not fully processing what he was saying or that she did not agree. He tested his hypothesis in several ways. First, as is standard with every patient, he took care either to summarize often during the session or to ask Sally to summarize. He also had her rate how much she believed the summary (e.g., "Sally, we've just been talking about the idea that you're not fully responsible for your father's unhappiness even though you did move far away. How much do you believe that now?").

The therapist further checked on Sally's understanding at different points during the session (e.g., "Is it clear to you why else your father might be reacting in this way? . . . Could you put it in your own words?"). The therapist also made sure to elicit feedback at the end of the session (e.g., "Anything I said today that bothered you? . . . Anything you think I didn't get quite right?"). Because he guessed that Sally might hesitate to give him negative feedback, he also asked very specifically for feedback about a *portion* of the session during which he suspected she might have had a negative reaction: "How about when I suggested that you might be able to be more assertive with your father? Did that bother you? . . . Do you think you would be able to tell me if it *had* bothered you?"

Finally, the therapist can try to uncover the existence of a problem at the next session. This investigation naturally falls into the portion of the session in which the therapist draws a bridge between the current session and the previous one. Sally's therapist, for example, listened to their therapy tape between sessions. Her tone of voice at a particular point on the tape prompted him to ask Sally about it at the next session: "Sally, I wonder how you felt about my asking you questions about your relationship with your father last week?" As the patient was noncommittal in her response, the therapist posed his concerns to her directly: "Did you feel I was pushing you too much or that you were being disloyal to your father?"

In summary, the therapist seeks to allay or to uncover problems within a therapy session by checking on the patient's understanding, by asking for feedback, and by raising suspected problems directly during the session itself or at the subsequent session. He may also ask the patient to complete a written evaluation of each session (see Chapter 3, Figure 3.3) which he can discuss at the next session.

The novice therapist, however, may be unaware of the existence of a problem in therapy and/or be less able to specify a problem precisely. He should solicit permission to audiotape therapy sessions to review on his own or (preferably) with an experienced cognitive therapist. Obtaining the patient's consent is usually not a problem if the therapist presents it as being to the patient's benefit (e.g., "Sally, I routinely tape my patient's sessions. Then I can listen to them between sessions if I think it'll help me plan therapy better. Sometimes, I play them to a colleague [or supervisor] to get feedback. Is that okay with you?").

The therapist may also uncover the existence of a problem by tracking the patient's progress. Having the patient complete objective tests such as the Beck Depression Inventory (see Appendix D) each week or having the patient rate her mood according to a 0–10 scale (see Chapter 3) at the beginning of each session can help both therapist and patient gauge progress. If the patient's symptoms fail to improve, the therapist can suggest this lack of progress as an agenda item and the two can collaborate in planning a more effective direction in therapy.

Finally, the therapist continually tries to put himself in the patient's shoes, to see how she views her world and to reveal what obstacles might inhibit her ability to take a more functional perspective of her difficulties (e.g., "If I were Sally, how would I feel during therapy? What would I think when my therapist said _____ or _____?").

CONCEPTUALIZING PROBLEMS

Having identified the existence of a problem, the therapist conceptualizes the level at which the problem occurred:

1. Is it merely a *technical problem*? For example, was a technique incorrectly employed or inappropriately selected?

> 2. Is it a more *complex problem with the session as a whole?* For example, did the therapist correctly identify a dysfunctional cognition but then fail to intervene effectively?
> 3. Is there an *ongoing problem across several sessions?* For example, has there been a breakdown in collaboration?

Typically, problems occur in one or more of the following categories:

> 1. Diagnosis, conceptualization, and treatment planning.
> 2. Therapeutic alliance.
> 3. Structure and/or pace of the session.
> 4. Socialization of the patient.
> 5. Dealing with automatic thoughts.
> 6. Accomplishing therapeutic goals in and across sessions.
> 7. Patient's processing of the session content.

The following questions can help the therapist and supervisor specify the nature of a therapeutic problem. Then they can formulate, prioritize, and select one or more specific objectives to focus on.

Diagnosis, Conceptualization, and Treatment Planning

Diagnosis
1. Do I have a correct diagnosis on the five axes according to the latest DSM?
2. If applicable, are the primary and secondary diagnoses in the appropriate order?
3. Could the patient be suffering from an undiagnosed organic problem?
4. Is a medication consult indicated for this patient?

Conceptualization
1. Do I have a concrete, sound conceptualization?
2. Can I express in words and on paper (perhaps using the Cognitive Conceptualization Diagram) how the patient's reactions (automatic thoughts, emotions, behaviors, physiological responses) to current situations relate to her history, beliefs, and strategies?
3. Have I continually refined my conceptualization as I got new data?
4. Have I shared my conceptualization with the patient at strategically appropriate times?
5. If so, does the conceptualization make sense and "ring true" to the patient?

Treatment Planning

1. Have I initially oriented therapy toward the primary Axis I disorder?
2. Have I varied standard cognitive therapy for this patient's Axis I (and/or Axis II) disorder(s)? Have I used my conceptualization in planning how to tailor therapy for this particular patient?
3. Have I addressed the need for a major life change if it has become apparent that improvement via therapy alone is unlikely? (This might be the case, for example, when the patient is in an abusive relationship, when her living conditions are intolerable, or when her job is quite deleterious to her.)
4. Have I appropriately planned for necessary skills training?
5. Have I included family members in therapy when appropriate?

Therapeutic Alliance

Collaboration

1. Have the patient and I been truly *collaborating*? Are we functioning as a team? Are we both working hard? Do we both feel responsible for progress?
2. Are we jointly making therapeutic decisions? Have we successfully negotiated issues such as homework, allotment of time for agenda items, etc.? Have we been covering the problems that are of most concern to the patient?
3. Have I guided the patient to an appropriate level of compliance and control in the therapy session?
4. Have we agreed on her goals and my goals for therapy?
5. Have I provided the rationale for my interventions and homework assignments?

Patient's Feedback

1. Do I regularly ask the patient for feedback about the session?
2. Do I encourage her to express and then evaluate her doubts?
3. Do I monitor the patient's affect during the session and ask for automatic thoughts when her affect shifts?

Patient's View of Therapy

1. Does the patient have a positive view of therapy and of me?
2. Does she believe, at least somewhat, that therapy can help her?
3. Does she see me as competent, collaborative, and caring?

Therapist's Reactions

1. Do I care about this patient? Does my caring come across to her?

2. Do I feel competent to help this patient? Does my sense of competence come across to her?
3. Do I have negative thoughts about this patient or about myself with respect to this patient? Have I evaluated and responded to these thoughts?
4. Do I see problems in the therapeutic alliance as an opportunity for growth versus assigning blame?
5. Do I project a realistically upbeat and optimistic view of how therapy can help?

Structuring and Pacing the Therapy Session

Agenda
1. Have we set a specific agenda?
2. Have we done so collaboratively with both of us contributing?
3. Have we set the agenda quickly?
4. Has the patient named her agenda topic(s) in a few words rather than providing a long description?
5. Has the patient named the agenda topic instead of discussing the item itself?
6. Have we prioritized the agenda topics?
7. Have we collaboratively set time allotments for each topic?
8. Have we collaboratively determined which topic to discuss first?

Pacing
1. Have I monitored how we have spent our therapy time?
2. Have we allotted and spent an appropriate amount of time for the standard session elements: mood check, brief review of the week, setting the agenda, homework review, discussion of agenda topic(s), periodic summaries, feedback?
3. When an agenda topic or session element exceeded its time allotment, did we collaboratively determine whether to continue or turn to the next item?
4. If important topics arose that were not part of the original agenda, did we collaboratively decide what to do?
5. Did we spend too much time on unproductive discourse?
6. Did I appropriately and gently interrupt the patient to guide our discussions toward more fruitful issues?
7. Did we leave enough time at the end of the session to summarize the most important points, to allow the patient to write down new conclusions, to ensure that the patient understood and agreed with the new homework assignment, to elicit feedback in a nonperfunctory way, and to respond to the feedback?

8. Did I pace the session in such a way as to deactivate core beliefs and diminish the patient's negative emotions so she did not leave the session feeling unduly distressed?

Socializing the Patient to Cognitive Therapy

Cognitive Model
1. Does the patient understand and agree with the cognitive model?
2. Does she understand that distorted thinking is a symptom of her disorder?
3. Does she believe that her thoughts about a situation may be distorted?
4. Does she realize that distorted thinking influences her mood and behaviors in dysfunctional ways?
5. Does she believe that she can feel better and behave more adaptively if she evaluates and modifies her dysfunctional thinking?
6. Does she believe she is capable of change?
7. Is she willing to make changes?

Expectations
1. What are the patient's expectations of herself and me in therapy?
2. Does she believe she should be able to solve her problems quickly and easily?
3. Does she expect me to solve her problems for her?
4. Does she believe her problems can be solved?
5. Does she understand her role and her responsibilities in therapy?
6. Does she understand that she needs to take an active role?
7. Does she collaborate easily?
8. Does she understand that she needs to learn certain tools and skills and to use them?
9. Does she fear solving current problems because then she will have to tackle other problems (such as career choice, relationship decisions, etc.)?

Problem-Solving Orientation
1. Does the patient specify problems to work on?
2. Do we actively work to solve problems rather than just airing problems?
3. Has she set specific goals? Are her goals realistic?
4. Does she understand how the work of each session is related to these goals?
5. Is she trying to change someone else rather than herself?

Homework
1. Does the patient do homework thoroughly?
2. Does she see it as optional or necessary?
3. Does she do homework only to please me?
4. Does she understand how homework relates to the work of the therapy session and to her overall goals?
5. Does she think about our therapy work throughout the week?
6. Has homework been well designed around her key issues?

Dealing with Automatic Thoughts

Identifying and Selecting Key Automatic Thoughts
1. Have we identified the actual words and/or images that went through the patient's mind when she was distressed?
2. Did we identify all the relevant automatic thoughts?
3. Did we select one thought to evaluate at a time?
4. Did we choose a thought that was associated with emotional distress?
5. Did we choose a thought that was either dysfunctional or likely to be distorted?
6. Did we choose a thought that, when modified, was likely to help the patient reach her goal or solve a problem? That is, was the thought an important one?

Responding to Automatic Thoughts
1. Did we not only identify a key automatic thought but also evaluate and respond to it?
2. Did I avoid assuming *a priori* that the thought was distorted? Did I avoid merely persuading the patient her thinking was wrong instead of collaboratively evaluating the thought?
3. Did I primarily use questioning?
4. If one line of questioning was ineffective, did I try other ways?
5. Did I avoid an overly challenging and/or persuasive stance?
6. Having collaboratively formulated an alternative response, did I check to see how much the patient believed it? Did her emotional distress decrease?
7. If needed, did we try other techniques to reduce the patient's distress? If needed, did we mark this automatic thought for future work?

Maximizing Cognitive Change
1. Did the patient write down her new, more functional understandings?
2. Did we identify the cognitive distortion?

3. Did we explore whether the patient had made similar distortions in the past and predict possible distortions of this type in the future?

Accomplishing Therapeutic Goals in and across Sessions

Identifying Overall Therapeutic Goals and Session-by-Session Objectives
1. Have I appropriately expressed these goals to the patient (if she has not already set them for herself)? Does she agree with these goals (e.g., to learn to do Dysfunctional Thought Records, to change how she spends her time, and to use a variety of anxiety-reduction techniques)?
2. Have I broken down these goals into intermediate objectives according to the phase of therapy we are in?
3. Do I use these objectives to guide the agenda setting?
4. Do I use the patient's agenda items to accomplish my objectives whenever appropriate?
5. In a given session, have I helped the patient identify an important problem on which to focus?
6. Is the problem appropriate to the patient's level of functioning and to her stage of therapy? For example, is the problem too closely tied to a rigid belief for progress to be made at this specific session?
7. Do we devote time to both problem-solving *and* cognitive restructuring?
8. Do we work on both behavioral change *and* cognitive change for homework?

Maintaining a Consistent Focus
1. Do I use guided discovery to help the patient identify relevant beliefs?
2. Can I state which beliefs of the patient are most central and which are more peripheral? Does the patient agree?
3. Do I consistently explore the relationship of new problems to the central beliefs, or do we jump from one problem to the next or from one dysfunctional belief to the next without relating them to the overall conceptualization?
4. Are we doing consistent, sustained work on the patient's central beliefs at each session instead of only crisis intervention?
5. When discussing childhood events, do I help the patient translate her interpretations into beliefs?
6. Do I help her see how these beliefs relate to her current problems?

Interventions
1. Do I choose interventions based on both my goals for the session and the patient's agenda?
2. Can I clearly state to myself both the patient's dysfunctional belief and a more functional belief toward which I am guiding her?
3. Did I check how distressed the patient felt and/or how strongly she endorsed an automatic thought or belief both before and after an intervention so I could judge how successful the intervention was?
4. If an intervention was relatively unsuccessful, did I switch gears and try another approach?
5. Did I conceptualize why the intervention was relatively unsuccessful? Was it due more to the selection or implementation of the technique or to the strength of the patient's dysfunctional thinking?

Patient's Processing of the Session Content

Monitoring Patient's Understanding
1. Have I summarized (or asked the patient to summarize) frequently during the session?
2. Have I asked the patient whether the content is clear and/or asked her to state conclusions in her own words?
3. Have I been alert for nonverbal signs of confusion or disagreement?

Conceptualizing Problems in Understanding
1. Have I checked out my hypotheses with the patient?
2. If she has difficulty understanding what I am trying to express, is it due to a mistake I have made?
3. Is a difficulty in understanding related to the level of complexity? To my lack of concreteness? To my vocabulary? To the amount of material I am presenting in one chunk or in one session?
4. Is a difficulty in understanding due to the patient's level of emotional distress in the therapy session? To distractions? To automatic thoughts the patient is having in session?

Maximizing Consolidation of Learning
1. What have I done to ensure that the patient will remember key parts of the therapy session during the week and even after therapy has ended?
2. Has the patient recorded key points in writing or on an audiotape?

STUCK POINTS

At times, a patient may feel better in individual sessions but does not seem to be making progress over the course of several sessions. The experienced therapist, in lieu of the preceding questions, may first wish to rule in or rule out five key problem areas. Having determined that he has a correct diagnosis, conceptualization, and treatment plan tailored for the patient's disorder (and has correctly employed techniques), the therapist assesses the following, alone or with a consultant:

1. Do the patient and I have a solid *therapeutic alliance*?
2. Do we both have a clear idea of the *patient's goals* for therapy? Is she committed to working toward her goals?
3. Does the patient truly believe the *cognitive model*—that her thinking influences her mood and behavior, that her thinking at times is dysfunctional, and that evaluating and responding to dysfunctional thinking positively affect how she feels emotionally and how she behaves?
4. Is the patient *socialized* to cognitive therapy—does she contribute to the agenda, collaboratively work toward solving problems, do homework, provide feedback to the therapist?
5. Is the patient's *biology* (e.g., illness, medication side effects, or inadequate level of medication) or her *external environment* (e.g., an abusive partner, an extremely demanding job, or an intolerable level of poverty or crime in her environment) interfering with our work?

REMEDIATING PROBLEMS IN THERAPY

Depending on the identified problem, the therapist might consider the advisability of one or more of the following steps:

1. Doing a more in-depth diagnostic evaluation.
2. Referring the patient for a physical or neuropsychological examination.
3. Refining the conceptualization of the patient in writing and checking it out with the patient.
4. Reading more about the treatment of the patient's Axis I (and Axis II) disorder(s).
5. Seeking specific feedback from the patient about her experience of therapy and of the therapist.
6. Reestablishing the patient's goals for therapy (and possibly examining the advantages and disadvantages of accomplishing them).

7. Identifying and responding to the therapist's own automatic thoughts about this patient or about his skill as a therapist.
8. Reviewing the cognitive model with the patient and eliciting any doubts or misunderstandings she may have.
9. Reviewing the treatment plan with the patient (and eliciting her concerns or doubts about it).
10. Reviewing the patient's responsibilities (and eliciting her reactions).
11. Emphasizing setting and reviewing homework in session and accomplishment of homework throughout the week.
12. Working consistently on *key* automatic thoughts, beliefs, and behaviors across sessions.
13. Checking on the patient's understanding of session content and having her record the most important points.
14. Based on the patient's needs and preferences, changing (in one direction or the other) the pace or structure of the session, the amount or difficulty of material covered, the degree of empathy expressed by the therapist, the degree to which the therapist is didactic or persuasive, and/or the relative focus on problem-solving.

The therapist should monitor his own thoughts and mood when seeking to conceptualize and remediate problems in therapy because his cognitions may at times interfere with problem-solving. It is likely that all therapists, at least occasionally, have negative thoughts about patients, the therapy, and/or themselves as therapists. Typical therapist assumptions that interfere with making changes to the therapy format include these:

"If I interrupt the patient, she'll think I'm controlling her."
"If I structure the session with an agenda, I'll miss something important."
"If I tape-record a session, I'll be too self-conscious."
"If my patient gets annoyed with me, she'll drop out of therapy."

Finally, the therapist who encounters a problem in therapy has a choice. He can catastrophize about the problem and/or blame himself or the patient. Alternatively, he can turn the problem into an opportunity to refine his skills of conceptualization and treatment planning and to improve his technical expertise and his ability to vary therapy in accordance with the specific needs of each individual patient.

PROGRESSING AS A COGNITIVE THERAPIST

This chapter briefly outlines steps to initiate the practice of standard cognitive therapy. As mentioned in Chapter 1, you are urged to gain experience with the basic techniques of cognitive therapy by practicing them yourself before doing so with patients. (See Appendix D for information on obtaining patient worksheets, tests, and pamphlets.) Trying the techniques yourself allows you to correct difficulties in application and putting yourself in the patient's role affords you the opportunity to identify obstacles (practical or psychological) that interfere with carrying out assignments. At a minimum, if you wish to become proficient in cognitive therapy, you should do the following (if you have not done so already):

1. Monitor your moods and identify your automatic thoughts when you experience dysphoria.

2. Write down your automatic thoughts. If you skip this step, you are depriving yourself of the opportunity to discover potential obstacles that your patients may have in writing down *their* thoughts: lack of opportunity, motivation, time, energy, and hope. When doing such things as assigning homework in session, you can then make a rapid comparison between yourself and the patient. You think, "Would I have difficulty doing this assignment? What would I need to become motivated? Is this assignment reasonable? What would get in the way of my doing it? Would I understand it if it had been presented to me that way? Do I need to present it in a more step-by-step fashion?" In other words, your progress as a cognitive therapist is facilitated if you bring an understanding of yourself and human nature in general to therapy.

3. Identify your automatic thoughts that interfere with carrying out

step 2 above. Thoughts such as "I don't have to write my automatic thoughts down," or "I know this stuff. I can get by with doing this in my head," are likely to impede your progress. A good adaptive response would acknowledge the partial truth of these thoughts but emphasize the advantages of behaving otherwise: "It's true that I can probably get by without using cognitive therapy tools on myself. But it's also true that I will probably learn considerably *more* if I go ahead and write things down. I'll better understand why my patients have difficulty if I myself go through the same process first to see what it feels like and spot potential trouble spots. What's the big deal anyway? It'll only take a couple of minutes."

4. Once you have become proficient at identifying your automatic thoughts and emotions, start doing one Dysfunctional Thought Record (DTR) a day when you notice your mood changing. Realize, however, that if your thoughts are not very distorted, or if you tend automatically to respond adaptively to your thoughts in your head, doing a DTR may not lead to much of a decrease in dysphoria. (Remember that the cognitive therapist does not try to *eliminate* negative emotion; he just tries to reduce *dysfunctional* degrees of emotion.) However, whether or not you personally benefit from doing DTRs, practicing doing them will sharpen your skill in teaching your patients to do them.

5. Fill out the bottom half of the Cognitive Conceptualization Diagram using three typical situations in which you felt dysphoric. If you have difficulty specifying the situation, identifying your thoughts or emotions, or uncovering the meaning of your thoughts, reread the relevant chapters in this book.

6. Continue to fill in the top half of the Cognitive Conceptualization Diagram. When you feel distressed, see whether there is a theme in the category of unlovability or helplessness underneath. Once you have identified a core belief, fill in the other boxes.

7. Next, using a core belief identified in the prior exercises, fill out a Core Belief Worksheet. Examine your interpretation of situations to determine whether you are distorting evidence to support a negative core belief and/or if you are ignoring or discounting evidence contrary to this core belief. Note: This exercise may not affect your belief system if you have positive, counterbalancing beliefs that are continuously activated, but completing the worksheet will at least make you more familiar with it and more likely to use it effectively with others.

8. Try doing some other basic techniques: activity monitoring and scheduling, positive self-statement logs, responding to spontaneous imagery, acting "as if," the problem-solving worksheet, writing and reading coping cards, making functional comparisons of the self, and writing down advantages and disadvantages when making a decision.

9. Having used some of the fundamental conceptual and treatment

tools yourself, choose a straightforward, uncomplicated patient for your first attempt at cognitive therapy. If you select a difficult patient, the standard treatment as described in this book may be inappropriate (see Chapter 16). The ideal patient for a first cognitive therapy experience is one who has a simple unipolar depression, generalized anxiety disorder, or adjustment disorder, with no diagnosis on Axis II. It is preferable to start with a new patient, rather than one whom you have been treating for a time using a different therapeutic orientation. It is also desirable to treat this patient according to the guidelines presented in this book, in as pure a fashion as possible. A note of caution: Therapists who are experienced in a different modality are often tempted to fall back on previously acquired skills that hinder cognitive therapy treatment.

10. Obtain written consent for audio- or videotaping of therapy sessions. Review of therapy tapes, either by yourself or with a colleague or supervisor, is essential to progress. An indispensable tool for evaluating your tapes is the Cognitive Therapy Scale and Manual (see Appendix D). It is used extensively by cognitive therapy supervisors to help trainees evaluate their work and plan for improvement.

11. Continue throughout this process to read more about cognitive therapy; consult the reading lists in Appendices B and C. Be sure to read pamphlets, articles, or books that are intended for patients so you will be able to suggest appropriate bibliotherapeutic readings to them.

12. Seek out opportunities for training and supervision, either locally or through the Beck Institute for Cognitive Therapy and Research (see Appendix D).

13. Finally, consider joining and attending conferences of the International Association for Cognitive Psychotherapy, the Association for Advancement of Behavior Therapy, the European Association of Behavior and Cognitive Therapy, or local associations of cognitive and behavioral therapy. See Appendix D for the addresses of these organizations.

CASE SUMMARY WORKSHEET

Therapist's name: *J. Beck*   **Patient's name:** *Sally R.*   **Date:** 2/10

I. Identifying information

Sally is an 18-year-old Caucasian female college student, living in a freshman dorm with one roommate.

II. Diagnoses (DSM-IV)

Axis I: *Major depression, single episode, moderate* 296.22

Axis II: *No personality disorder*

Axis III: *No physical disorders or conditions*

Axis IV: *Severity of psychosocial stressors: mild (leaving home for first time)*

Axis V: *Global assessment of functioning: current* 60; *past year* 85

III. Objective scores

	Intake	Sess. no.	Sess. no.	Sess. no.	Sess. no.	Sess. no.	Sess. no.	Last Sess.
BDI*	27							
BAI*	15							
BHS*	15							
Other								

General trend of scores:

*BDI, Beck Depression Inventory; BAI, Beck Anxiety Inventory; HS, Beck Hopelessness Scale.

IV. Presenting problems and current functioning

Complaints of depression, anxiety, difficulties in concentration, social withdrawal, increased sleep, self-criticism. Attending classes but difficulty studying and completing work. Avoiding problems with roommate.

V. Developmental profile

A. History (family, social, educational, medical, psychiatric, vocational)

Younger of two children in intact family.
Always had several friends.
Average to good grades in school; some anxiety over grades.
No significant medical problems; no prior psychiatric history; good part-time work record last year.

B. Relationships (parents, siblings, peers, authority figures, significant others)

Mother was (and is) highly critical of Sally; father is/was more supportive but not physically present a lot (demanding job).
Got along well with brother despite 5-year age difference.
Feared harsh teachers.

C. Significant events and traumas

Parents argued a lot.
Harsh teacher in second grade (I was scared the whole year).
Subtle trauma: criticism by mother.
Self-criticism for not measuring up to brother.

VI. Cognitive profile

A. The cognitive model as applied to this patient

1. Typical current problems/problematic situations:

Studying and writing papers.
Volunteering in class and taking tests.
Social withdrawal.
Lack of assertiveness with roommate, professors.
Spending too much time in bed.

2. Typical automatic thoughts, affect, and behaviors in these situations:

I can't do this; I'm such a failure; I'll never make it here. → *Sad*
What if I flunk the test; what if the teaching assistant won't help me, I might flunk out. → *Anxious*
I should be doing more, doing better. → *Guilty*

B. Core beliefs

I'm inadequate/incompetent.

C. Conditional beliefs

If I don't do great, then I've failed.
If I fail at school, I'm a failure as a person.
If I ask for help, I'm weak.

D. Rules (shoulds/musts applied to self/others)

I must work very hard.
I must live up to my potential.
I must excel.

VII. Integration and conceptualization of cognitive and developmental profiles

A. Formulation of self-concept and concepts of others

Sally saw herself as competent at some things but incompetent and inadequate at others. She overestimated others' (brother, friends) strengths and underestimated her own.

B. Interaction of life events and cognitive vulnerabilities

Sally has always been vulnerable to seeing herself as inadequate. Her highly critical mother reinforced her belief that she was inadequate. In addition, Sally continually compared herself unfavorably to her brother, who (because he was 5 years older) could do almost everything better than she could.

C. Compensatory and coping strategies

Holds high expectations for herself.
Works very hard.
Is hypervigilant for shortcomings.
Avoids seeking help.

D. Development and maintenance of current disorder

Depressive disorder was precipitated by leaving home for college and experiencing some initial difficulty in her courses. Anxiety probably interfered with efficient studying; then Sally became quite self-critical and dysphoric. As she withdrew from activities and friends, the lack of positive input contributed to her low mood.

VIII. Implications for therapy

A. Suitability for cognitive interventions (rate low, medium, or high; add comments, if applicable):

1. Psychological mindedness—*high*
2. Objectivity—*high*
3. Awareness—*medium/high*
4. Belief in cognitive model—*medium/high*
5. Accessibility and plasticity of automatic thoughts and beliefs—*medium*
6. Adaptiveness—*high*
7. Humor—*low (at intake)*

B. Personality organization: sociotropic versus autonomous

Higher in autonomy than sociotropy:

Places high value on achievement, sees asking for help as a weakness.

Medium in sociotropy; does value friendships, concerned about how others view her.

C. Patient's motivation, goals, and expectations for therapy

Very motivated, had only vague expectations for therapy but agrees with model of becoming her own therapist.

Goals:

Improve school grades

Decrease worry about tests

Meet more people

Join school activities and/or get part-time job

D. Therapist's goals

Decrease self-criticism.

Teach basic cognitive tools, DTR, etc.

Decrease time in bed.

Do problem-solving around studying, papers, tests.

E. Predicted difficulties and modifications of standard cognitive therapy

None.

A BASIC COGNITIVE THERAPY
READING LIST FOR THERAPISTS

BOOKS, CHAPTERS, AND JOURNAL ARTICLES

Beck, A. T. (1976). *Cognitive therapy and the emotional disorders.* New York: International Universities Press.

Beck, A. T. (1988). *Love is never enough.* New York: Harper & Row.

Beck, A. T. (1991). Cognitive therapy: A 30-year retrospective. *American Psychologist, 46,* 368–375.

Beck, A. T., & Emery, G. (with Greenberg, R. L.). (1985). *Anxiety disorders and phobias: A cognitive perspective.* New York: Basic Books.

Beck, A. T., Freeman, A., & Associates. (1990). *Cognitive therapy of personality disorders.* New York: Guilford Press.

Beck, A. T., Rush, A. J., Shaw, B. F., & Emery, G. (1979). *Cognitive therapy of depression.* New York: Guilford Press.

Beck, A. T., Wright, F. D., Newman, C. F., & Liese, B. S. (1993). *Cognitive therapy of substance abuse.* New York: Guilford Press.

Clark, D. M. (1989). Anxiety states: Panic and generalized anxiety. In K. Hawton, P. M. Salkovskis, J. Kirk, & D. M. Clark (Eds.), *Cognitive behaviour therapy for psychiatric problems: A practical guide* (pp. 52–96). Oxford: Oxford University Press.

Dattilio, F. M., & Padesky, C. A. (1990). *Cognitive therapy with couples.* Sarasota, FL: Professional Resource Exchange.

Edwards, D. J. A. (1989). Cognitive restructuring through guided imagery: Lessons from Gestalt therapy. In A. Freeman, K. M. Simon, L. E. Beutler, & H. Arkowitz (Eds.), *Comprehensive handbook of cognitive therapy* (pp. 283–298). New York: Plenum Press.

Epstein, N., Schlesinger, S. E., & Dryden, W. (1988). *Cognitive–behavioral therapy with families.* New York: Brunner/Mazel.

Fennell, M. J. V. (1989). Depression. In K. Hawton, P. M. Salkovskis, J. Kirk, &

D. M. Clark (Eds.), *Cognitive behaviour therapy for psychiatric problems: A practical guide* (169–234). Oxford: Oxford University Press.

Freeman, A. (Ed.). (1983). *Cognitive therapy with couples and groups.* New York: Plenum Press.

Freeman, A., & Dattilio, F. M. (Eds.). (1992). *Comprehensive casebook of cognitive therapy.* New York: Plenum Press.

Freeman, A., Pretzer, J., Fleming, B., & Simon, K. M. (1990). *Clinical applications of cognitive therapy.* New York: Plenum Press.

Freeman, A., Simon, K. M., Beutler, L. E., & Arkowitz, H. (Eds.). (1989). *Comprehensive handbook of cognitive therapy.* New York: Plenum Press.

Garner, D. M., & Bemis, K. M. (1985). Cognitive therapy for anorexia nervosa. In D. M. Garner & P. E. Garfinkel (Eds.), *Handbook of psychotherapy for anorexia nervosa and bulimia* (pp. 107–146). New York: Guilford Press.

Hawton, K., Salkovskis, P. M., Kirk, J., & Clark, D. M. (Eds.). (1989). *Cognitive behaviour therapy for psychiatric problems: A practical guide.* Oxford: Oxford University Press.

Hollon, S. D., & Beck, A. T. (1993). Cognitive and cognitive–behavioral therapies. In A. E. Bergin, & S. L. Garfield (Eds.), *Handbook of psychotherapy and behavior change: An empirical analysis* (4th ed., pp. 428–466). New York: Wiley.

Kuehlwein, K. T., & Rosen, H. (Eds.). (1993). *Cognitive therapies in action: Evolving innovative practice.* San Francisco: Jossey-Bass.

Layden, M. A., Newman, C. F., Freeman, A., & Morse, S. B. (1993). *Cognitive therapy of borderline personality disorder.* Needham Heights, MA: Allyn & Bacon.

McMullin, R. E. (1986). *Handbook of cognitive therapy techniques.* New York: W. W. Norton.

Persons, J. B. (1989). *Cognitive therapy in practice: A case formulation approach.* New York: W. W. Norton.

Safran, J. D., Vallis, T. M., Segal, Z. V., & Shaw, B. F. (1986). Assessment of core cognitive processes in cognitive therapy. *Cognitive Therapy and Research, 10,* 509–526.

Scott, J., Williams, J. M. G., & Beck, A. T. (Eds.). (1989). *Cognitive therapy in clinical practice: An illustrative casebook.* New York: Routledge.

Wright, J. H., & Beck, A. T. (in press). Cognitive therapy. In R. E. Hales, J. A. Talbott, & S. C. Yudofsky (Eds.), *The American Psychiatric Press textbook of psychiatry* (2nd ed.). Washington, DC: American Psychiatric Press.

Wright, J., Thase, M., Beck, A. T., & Ludgate, J. (Eds.). (1993). *Cognitive therapy with inpatients.* New York: Guilford Press.

Young, J. E. (1990). *Cognitive therapy for personality disorders: A schema-focused approach.* Sarasota, FL: Professional Resource Exchange.

JOURNALS

Cognitive and Behavioral Practice. Published by the Association for Advancement of Behavior Therapy.

Cognitive Therapy and Research. Published by Plenum Press, New York.

Journal of Cognitive Psychotherapy, an International Quarterly. Published by Springer, New York; also available through the IACP (see Appendix D).
The Behavior Therapist. Published by the Association for Advancement of Behavior Therapy, New York.

NEWSLETTER

International Association for Cognitive Psychotherapy Newsletter. Available from the IACP (see Appendix D).

COGNITIVE THERAPY READING LIST FOR PATIENTS (AND THERAPISTS)

Beck, A. T. (1988). *Love is never enough*. New York: Harper & Row.

Beck, A. T., & Greenberg, R. L. (1995). *Coping with depression* (rev. ed.). Bala Cynwyd, PA: Beck Institute for Cognitive Therapy and Research.

Beck, A. T., & Emery, G. (1995). *Coping with anxiety and panic* (rev. ed.). Bala Cynwyd, PA: Beck Institute for Cognitive Therapy and Research.

Bricker, D. C., & Young, J. E. (1991). *A client's guide to schema-focused cognitive therapy*. New York: Cognitive Therapy Center of New York.

Burns, D. D. (1980). *Feeling good: The new mood therapy*. New York: New American Library.

Burns, D. D. (1989). *The feeling good handbook: Using the new mood therapy in everyday life*. New York: William Morrow.

Greenberg, R. L., & Beck, A. T. (1995). *Panic attacks: How to cope, how to recover* (rev. ed.). Bala Cynwyd, PA: Beck Institute for Cognitive Therapy and Research.

Greenberger, D., & Padesky, C. (1995). *Mind over mood: A cognitive therapy treatment manual for clients*. New York: Guilford Press.

McKay, M., & Fanning, P. (1991). *Prisoners of belief*. Oakland, CA: New Harbinger.

McKay, M., & Fanning, P. (1987). *Self-esteem*. Oakland, CA: New Harbinger.

Morse, S. B., Morse, M., & Nackoul, K. (1992). *Cognitive principles and techniques: A video series and workbooks*. Albuquerque, NM: Creative Cognitive Therapy Productions.

Young, J. E., & Klosko, J. (1994). *Reinventing your life: How to break free of negative life patterns*. New York: Dutton.

COGNITIVE THERAPY RESOURCES

TRAINING PROGRAMS

The Beck Institute for Cognitive Therapy and Research in suburban Philadelphia offers intramural and extramural training programs.

> Beck Institute for Cognitive Therapy and Research
> GSB Building, Suite 700
> City Line and Belmont Avenues
> Bala Cynwyd, PA 19004-1610
> USA
> Phone: 610/664-3020 Fax: 610/664-4437

THERAPIST AND PATIENT MATERIALS

The following may be ordered from the Beck Institute at the above address:

> Patient pamphlets
> Worksheet packets
> Cognitive Therapy Rating Scale and Manual
> Books, videotapes, and audiotapes by Aaron T. Beck, M.D.
> Beck Institute Training Program Brochure
> Beck Institute Educational Catalog
> Information about the Cognitive Therapy Interactive Computer Program for Patients, developed by Jesse Wright, M.D., and Aaron T. Beck, M.D.

ASSESSMENT MATERIALS

The following scales and manuals may be ordered from The Psychological Corporation, 555 Academic Court, San Antonio, TX, 78204-9990, 1-800-228-0752:

> Beck Depression Inventory and Manual
> Beck Anxiety Inventory
> Beck Hopelessness Scale
> Beck Scale for Suicidal Ideation.

Beck Children's Inventories are in development and will be available in the future from The Psychological Corporation.

COGNITIVE THERAPY PROFESSIONAL ORGANIZATIONS

> International Association for Cognitive Psychotherapy
> Beck Institute for Cognitive Therapy
> GSB Building, Suite 700
> City Line and Belmont Avenues
> Bala Cynwyd, PA 19004-1610
> USA
> Phone: 610/664-3020 Fax: 610/664-4437

> Association for Advancement of Behavior Therapy
> 305 Seventh Avenue
> New York, NY 10001-6008
> USA
> Phone: 212/279-7970

> European Association of Behavior and Cognitive Therapy
> Rod Holland
> Northwick Park Hospital & Clinical Research Centre
> Watford Road, Harrow
> Middlesex HA13VJ
> United Kingdom

REFERENCES

Agras, W. S., Rossiter, E. M., Arnow, B., Schneider, J. A., Telch, C. F., Raeburn, S. D., Bruce, B., Perl, M., & Koran, L. M. (1992). Pharmacologic and cognitive–behavioral treatment for bulimia nervosa: A controlled comparison. *American Journal of Psychiatry, 149*, 82–87.

American Psychiatric Association. (1994). *Diagnostic and statistical manual of mental disorders* (4th ed.). Washington, DC: Author.

Arnkoff, D. B., & Glass, C. R. (1992). Cognitive therapy and psychotherapy integration. In D. K. Freedheim (Ed.), *History of psychotherapy: A century of change* (pp. 657–694). Washington, DC. American Psychological Association.

Barlow, D., Craske, M., Cerney, J. A., & Klosko, J. S. (1989). Behavioral treatment of panic disorder. *Behavior Therapy, 20*, 261–268.

Baucom, D., & Epstein, N. (1990). *Cognitive–behavioral marital therapy*. New York: Brunner/Mazel.

Baucom, D., Sayers, S., & Scher, T. (1990). Supplementary behavioral marital therapy with cognitive restructuring and emotional expressiveness training: An outcome investigation. *Journal of Consulting and Clinical Psychology, 58*, 636–645.

Beck, A. T. (1964). Thinking and depression: II. Theory and therapy. *Archives of General Psychiatry, 10*, 561–571.

Beck, A. T. (1976). *Cognitive therapy and the emotional disorders*. New York: International Universities Press.

Beck, A. T. (1987). Cognitive approaches to panic disorder: Theory and therapy. In S. Rachman, & J. Maser (Eds.), *Panic: Psychological perspectives* (pp. 91–109). Hillsdale, NJ: Erlbaum.

Beck, A. T. (1988). *Love is never enough*. New York: Harper & Row.

Beck, A. T. (in press). Cognitive aspects of personality disorders and their relation to syndromal disorders: A psychoevolutionary approach. In C. R. Cloninger (Ed.), *Personality and psychopathology*. Washington, DC: American Psychiatric Press.

Beck, A. T., & Emery, G. (with Greenberg, R. L.). (1985). *Anxiety disorders and phobias: A cognitive perspective*. New York: Basic Books.

Beck, A. T., Freeman, A., & Associates. (1990). *Cognitive therapy of personality disorders*. New York: Guilford Press.

Beck, A. T., & Greenberg, R. L. (1974). *Coping with depression*. Bala Cynwyd, PA: Beck Institute for Cognitive Therapy and Research.

Beck, A. T., & Steer, R. A. (1987). *Manual for the revised Beck Depression Inventory*. San Antonio, TX: The Psychological Corporation.

Beck, A. T., Rush, A. J., Shaw, B. F., & Emery, G. (1979). *Cognitive therapy of depression*. New York: Guilford Press.

Beck, A. T., Sokol, L., Clark, D. A., Berchick, R. J., & Wright, F. D. (1992). A crossover study of focused cognitive therapy for panic disorder. *American Journal of Psychiatry, 149*(6), 778–783.

Beck, A. T., Wright, F. W., Newman, C. F., & Liese, B. (1993). *Cognitive therapy of substance abuse*. New York: Guilford Press.

Bedrosian, R. C., & Bozicas, G. D. (1994). *Treating family of origin problems: A cognitive approach*. New York: Guilford Press.

Benson, H. (1975). *The relaxation response*. New York: Avon.

Beutler, L. E., Scogin, F., Kirkish, P., Schretlen, D., Corbishley, A., Hamblin, D., Meredity, K., Potter, R., Bamford, C. R., & Levenson, A. I. (1987). Group cognitive therapy and alprazalam in the treatment of depression in older adults. *Journal of Consulting and Clinical Psychology, 55*, 550–556.

Bowers, W. A. (1990). Treatment of depressed in- patients: Cognitive therapy plus medication, relaxation plus medication, and medication alone. *British Journal of Psychiatry, 156*, 73–78.

Bowers, W. A. (1993). Cognitive therapy for eating disorders. In J. Wright, M. Thase, A. T. Beck, & J. Ludgate (Eds.), *Cognitive therapy with inpatients* (pp. 337–356). New York: Guilford Press.

Burns, D. D. (1980). *Feeling good: The new mood therapy*. New York: Signet.

Burns, D. D. (1989). *The feeling good handbook: Using the new mood therapy in everyday life*. New York: Morrow.

Butler, G. (1989). Phobic disorders. In K. Hawton, P. M. Salkovskis, J. Kirk, & D. M. Clark (Eds.), *Cognitive–behavior therapy for psychiatric problems: A practical guide* (pp. 97–128). New York: Oxford University Press.

Butler, G., Fennell, M., Robson, D., & Gelder, M. (1991). Comparison of behavior therapy and cognitive–behavior therapy in the treatment of generalized anxiety disorder. *Journal of Consulting and Clinical Psychology, 59*, 167–175.

Casey, D. A., & Grant, R. W. (1993). Cognitive therapy with depressed elderly inpatients. In J. Wright, M. Thase, A. T. Beck, & J. Ludgate (Eds.), *Cognitive therapy with inpatients* (pp. 295–314). New York: Guilford Press.

Chadwick, P. D. J., & Lowe, C. F. (1990). Measurement and modification of delusional beliefs. *Journal of Consulting and Clinical Psychology, 58*, 225–232.

Clark, D. M. (1989). Anxiety states: Panic and generalized anxiety. In K. Hawton, P. M. Salkovskis, J. Kirk, & D. M. Clark (Eds.), *Cognitive–behavior therapy for psychiatric problems: A practical guide* (pp. 52–96). New York: Oxford University Press.

Clark, D. M., Salkovskis, P. M., Hackmann, A., Middleton, H., & Gelder, M. (1992). A comparison of cognitive therapy, applied relaxation, and imipramine in the treatment of panic disorder. *British Journal of Psychiatry, 164*, 759–769.

Dancu, C. V., & Foa, E. B. (1992). Posttraumatic stress disorder. In A. Freeman & F. M. Dattilio (Eds.), *Comprehensive casebook of cognitive therapy* (79–88). New York: Plenum Press.

Dattilio, F. M., & Padesky, C. A. (1990). *Cognitive therapy with couples.* Sarasota, FL: Professional Resource Exchange.

Davis, M., Eshelman, E. R., & McKay, M. (1988). *The relaxation and stress reduction workbook.* Oakland, CA: New Harbinger.

Dobson, K. S. (1989). A meta-analysis of the efficacy of cognitive therapy for depression. *Journal of Consulting and Clinical Psychology, 57,* 414–419.

Edwards, D. J. A. (1989). Cognitive restructuring through general guided imagery: Lessons from Gestalt therapy. In A. Freeman, K. M. Simon, L. E. Beutler, & H. Arkowitz (Eds.), *Comprehensive handbook of cognitive therapy* (pp. 283–297). New York: Plenum Press.

Ellis, A. (1962). *Reason and emotion in psychotherapy.* New York: Lyle Stuart.

Epstein, N., Schlesinger, S. E., & Dryden, W. (1988). *Cognitive–behavioral therapy with families.* New York: Brunner/Mazel.

Evans, J. M. G., Hollon, S. D., DeRubeis, R. J., Piasecki, J. M., Grove, W. M., Garvey, M. J., & Tuason, V. B. (1992). Differential relapse following cognitive therapy and pharmacology for depression. *Archives of General Psychiatry, 49,* 802–808.

Fairburn, C. G., & Cooper, P. J. (1989). Eating disorders. In K. Hawton, P. M. Salkovskis, J. Kirk, & D. M. Clark (Eds.), *Cognitive behavior therapy for psychiatric problems: A practical guide* (pp. 277–314). New York: Oxford University Press.

Fairburn, C. G., Jones, R., Peveler, R. C., Hope, R. A., & Doll, H. A. (1991). Three psychological treatments for bulimia nervosa: A comparative trial. *Archives of General Psychiatry, 48,* 463–469.

Freeman, A., & Dattilio, F. M. (Eds.). (1992). *Comprehensive casebook of cognitive therapy.* New York: Plenum Press.

Freeman, A., Pretzer, J., Fleming, B., & Simon, K. M. (1990). *Clinical applications of cognitive therapy.* New York: Plenum Press.

Freeman, A., Schrodt, G., Gilson, M., & Ludgate, J. (1993). Group cognitive therapy with inpatients. In J. Wright, M. Thase, A. T. Beck, & J. Ludgate (Eds.), *Cognitive therapy with inpatients* (pp. 121–153). New York: Guilford Press.

Freeman, A., Simon, K. M., Beutler, L. E., & Arkowitz, M. (Eds.). (1989). *Comprehensive handbook of cognitive therapy.* New York: Plenum Press.

Fremouw, W. J., dePerczel, N., & Ellis, T. E. (1990). *Suicide risk: Assessment and response.* New York: Pergamon Press.

Garner, D. M., & Bemis, K. M. (1985). Cognitive therapy for anorexia nervosa. In D. M. Garner & P. E. Garfinkel (Eds.), *Handbook of psychotherapy for anorexia nervosa and bulimia* (pp. 107–146). New York: Guilford Press.

Garner, D. M., Rockert, W., Davis, R., Garner, M. V., Olmstead, M. P., & Eagle, M. (1993). Comparison of cognitive–behavioral and supportive–expressive therapy for bulimia nervosa. *American Journal of Psychiatry, 150,* 37–46.

Gelernter, C. S., Uhde, T. W., Cimbolic, P., Arnkoff, D. B., Vittone, B. J., Tancer, M. E., & Bartko, J. J. (1991). Cognitive–behavioral and pharmacological treatments of social phobia: A controlled study. *Archives of General Psychiatry, 48,* 938–945.

Goldstein, A., & Stainback, B. (1987). *Overcoming agoraphobia: Conquering fear of the outside world.* New York: Viking Penguin.

Greenberger, D., & Padesky, C. (1995). *Mind over mood: A cognitive therapy treatment manual for clients.* New York: Guilford Press.

Goldstein, A., & Stainback, B. (1987). *Overcoming agoraphobia: Conquering fear of the outside world.* New York: Viking Penguin.

Guidano, V. F., & Liotti, G. (1983). *Cognitive processes and emotional disorders: A structural approach to psychotherapy.* New York: Guilford Press.

Heimberg, R. G. (1990). Cognitive behavior therapy (for social phobia). In A. S. Bellack, & M. Hersen (Eds.), *Comparative handbook of treatments for adult disorders* (pp. 203–218). New York: Wiley.

Heimberg, R. G., Dodge, C. S., Hope, D. A., Kennedy, C. R., Zollo, L. J., & Becker, R. E. (1990). Cognitive behavioral group treatment for social phobia: Comparison with a credible placebo control. *Cognitive Therapy and Research, 14,* 1–23.

Hollon, S. D., & Beck, A. T. (1993). Cognitive and cognitive–behavioral therapies. In A. E. Bergin & S.L. Garfield (Eds.), *Handbook of psychotherapy and behavior change: An empirical analysis* (4th ed., pp. 428–466). New York: Wiley.

Hollon, S. D., DeRubeis, R. J., & Seligman, M. E. P. (1992). Cognitive therapy and the prevention of depression. *Applied and Preventive Psychiatry, 1,* 89–95.

Jacobson, E. (1974). *Progressive relaxation.* Chicago: University of Chicago Press, Midway Reprint.

Kingdon, D. G., & Turkington, D. (1994). *Cognitive–behavioral therapy of schizophrenia.* New York: Guilford Press.

Knell, S. M. (1993). *Cognitive–behavioral play therapy.* Northvale, NJ: Jason Aronson.

Layden, M. A., Newman, C. F., Freeman, A., & Morse, S. B. (1993). *Cognitive therapy of borderline personality disorder.* Needham Heights, MA: Allyn & Bacon.

Lazarus, A. (1976). *Multimodal behavior therapy.* New York: Springer.

Mahoney, M. (1991). *Human change processes: The scientific foundations of psychotherapy.* New York: Basic Books.

Marlatt, G. A., & Gordon, J. R. (Eds.). (1985). *Relapse prevention: Maintenance strategies in the treatment of additive behaviors.* New York: Guilford Press.

McKay, M., & Fanning, P. (1991). *Prisoners of belief.* Oakland, CA: New Harbinger.

McMullin, R. E. (1986). *Handbook of cognitive therapy techniques.* New York: W. W. Norton.

Meichenbaum, D. (1977). *Cognitive–behavior modification: An integrative approach.* New York: Plenum Press.

Miller, I. W., Norman, W. H., Keitner, G. I., Bishop, S. B., & Dow, M. G. (1989). Cognitive–behavioral treatment of depressed inpatients. *Behavior Therapy, 20,* 25–47.

Miller, P. (1991). The application of cognitive therapy to chronic pain. In T. M. Vallis, J. L. Howes, & P. C. Miller (Eds.), *The challenge of cognitive therapy: Application to nontraditional populations* (pp. 159–182). New York: Plenum Press.

Morse, S. B., Morse, M., & Nackoul, K. (1992). *Cognitive principles and techniques: A video series and workbooks*. Albuquerque, NM: Creative Cognitive Therapy Productions.

Niemeyer, R. A., & Feixas, G. (1990). The role of homework and skill acquisition in the outcome of group cognitive therapy for depression. *Behavior Therapy, 21*(3), 281–292.

Overholser, J. C. (1993a). Elements of the Socratic method: I. Systematic questioning. *Psychotherapy, 30,* 67–74.

Overholser, J. C. (1993b). Elements of the Socratic method: II. Inductive reasoning. *Psychotherapy, 30,* 75–85.

Palmer, A. G., Williams, H., & Adams, M. (1994). *Cognitive behavioral therapy in a group for bipolar patients*. (Manuscript submitted for publication).

Parrott, C. A., & Howes, J. L. (1991). The application of cognitive therapy to post-traumatic stress disorder. In T. M. Vallis, J. L. Howes, & P. C. Miller (Eds.), *The challenge of cognitive therapy: Applications to nontraditional populations* (pp. 85–109). New York: Plenum Press.

Perris, C., Ingelson, U., & Johnson, D. (1993). Cognitive therapy as a general framework in the treatment of psychotic patients. In K. T. Kuehlwein & H. Rosen (Eds.), *Cognitive therapy in action: Evolving innovative practice* (pp. 379–402). San Francisco: Jossey-Bass.

Persons, J. B. (1989). *Cognitive therapy in practice*. New York: W. W. Norton.

Persons, J. B., Burns, D. D., & Perloff, J. M. (1988). Predictors of dropout and outcome in cognitive therapy for depression in a private practice setting. *Cognitive Therapy and Research, 12,* 557–575.

Rosen, H. (1988). The constructivist–development paradigm. In R. A. Dorfman (Ed.), *Paradigms of clinical social work* (pp. 317–355). New York: Brunner/Mazel.

Rush, A. J., Beck, A. T., Kovacs, M., & Hollon, S. D. (1977). Comparative efficacy of cognitive therapy and pharmacotherapy in the treatment of depressed outpatients. *Cognitive Therapy and Research, 1*(1), 17–37.

Safran, J. D., Vallis, T. M., Segal, Z. V., & Shaw, B. F. (1986). Assessment of core cognitive processes in cognitive therapy. *Cognitive Therapy and Research, 10,* 509–526.

Salkovskis, P. M., & Kirk, J. (1989). Obsessional disorders. In K. Hawton, P. M. Salkovskis, J. Kirk, & D. M. Clark (Eds.), *Cognitive-behavior therapy for psychiatric problems: A practical guide* (pp. 129–168). New York: Oxford University Press.

Scott, J., Williams, J. M. G., & Beck, A. T. (Eds.). (1989). *Cognitive therapy in clinical practice: An illustrative casebook*. New York: Routledge.

Thase, M. E., Bowler, K., & Harden, T. (1991). Cognitive behavior therapy of endogenous depression: Part 2. Preliminary findings in 16 unmedicated inpatients. *Behavior Therapy, 22,* 469–477.

Thompson, L. W., Davies, R., Gallagher, D., & Krantz, S. E. (1986). Cognitive therapy with older adults. In T. L. Bring (Ed.), *Clinical gerontology: A guide to assessment and intervention* (pp. 245–279). New York: Haworth Press.

Turk, D. C., Meichenbaum, D., & Genest, M. (1983). *Pain and behavioral medicine: A cognitive-behavioral perspective*. New York: Guilford Press.

Warwick, H. M. C., & Salkovskis, P. M. (1989). Hypochondriasis. In J. Scott, M.

G. Williams, & A. T. Beck (Eds.), *Cognitive therapy in clinical practice: An illustrative casebook* (pp. 50–77). London: Routledge.

Weissman, A. N., & Beck, A. T. (1978). *Development and validation of the Dysfunctional Attitude Scale: A preliminary investigation.* Paper presented at the Annual Meeting of the American Educational Research Association, Toronto, Canada.

Woody, G. E., Luborsky, L., McClellan, A. T., O'Brien, C. P., Beck, A. T., Blaine, J., Herman, I., & Hole, A. (1983). Psychotherapy for opiate addicts: Does it help? *Archives of General Psychiatry, 40,* 1081–1086.

Young, J. E. (1990). *Cognitive therapy for personality disorders: A schema focused approach.* Sarasota, FL: Professional Resources Exchange.

Young, J. E., & Klosko, J. (1994). *Reinventing your life: How to break free of negative life patterns.* New York: Dutton Press.

INDEX